THIS IS CANCER

THIS IS CANCER

Everything You Need to Know,
From the Waiting Room to the Bedroom

LAURA HOLMES HADDAD

SEAL PRESS

Seal Press
An imprint of Perseus Books,
A Hachette Book Group company
1700 Fourth Street
Berkeley, California
sealpress.com

978-1-58005-626-7

Library of Congress Cataloging-in-Publication Data

Names: Haddad, Laura Holmes, author.
Title: This is cancer : everything you need to know, from the waiting room to
    the bedroom / by Laura Holmes Haddad.
Description: Berkeley, California : Seal Press, [2016]
Identifiers: LCCN 2016026471 | ISBN 9781580056267 (paperback)
Subjects: LCSH: Haddad, Laura Holmes,—Health. |
    Breast—Cancer—Patients—Biography. | Women—Health and
    hygiene—Popular
        works. | Cancer—Popular works. | BISAC: HEALTH & FITNESS /
Diseases /
        Cancer. | SELF-HELP / Motivational & Inspirational. | HEALTH &
FITNESS /
    Women's Health.
Classification: LCC RC280.B8 H33 2016 | DDC 362.19699/4490092 [B]
    —dc23
LC record available at https://lccn.loc.gov/2016026471

10 9 8 7 6 5 4 3 2 1

Cover design by Erin Seaward-Hiatt
Interior design by Domini Dragoone
Printed in the United States of America

To Penelope and Roman,
who inspire me every day;

To Lesley,
for your exquisite fight plan;

and to Mark Moasser, MD,
for never giving up on me.

When you look ahead it may seem too hard.
Look again.
Always look again.

—Mary Anne Radmacher

CONTENTS

- My Doctor Is God, My Doctor Is Mortal
- Nurses: The Good, the Bad, and Everything in Between
- Paperwork: Passport for Cancer Patients
- Waiting Rooms: The Holding Tanks
- Cancerspeak, Part 1: A Translation Guide
- The Cost of Cancer (Literally): Medical Bills, Fees, and Finances
- First Opinion
- Second Opinion
- Off the Clock: Work and Cancer
- Journals, Emails, Blogs, and Other Public Airings
- Friends to Surround Yourself With
- Think Big (But Small)

- Scans
- Pokes and Pricks
- Cancerspeak, Part 2: A Guide to Medical Terms
  You Will Hear Over and Over (and Over Again)

PART 3: SURVIVAL

PART 4:

PART 5:

AUTHOR'S NOTE

This book is intended as a guide for cancer patients and care-givers, based on my own experiences as a young-ish breast cancer patient. It has been reviewed by an oncologist for spelling and clarification, but any mistakes are entirely my own. It is not intended to replace medical care; rather, it is a supplement to help you navigate the world of cancer.

INTRODUCTION

I am a Stage IV inflammatory breast cancer survivor. I went from perfectly healthy (lots of yoga, lots of broccoli) to not feeling great to being told I had an extensive tumor in my left breast and cancer that had spread to my lymph nodes and potentially a rib. I was given roughly three to five years to live, all at the age of thirty-seven. With the help of an incredibly diligent family and a team of brilliant doctors and a tiny green chemotherapy clinical trial drug, I'm still here. It is not an exaggeration to say it's a miracle that I'm alive. I am a survivor, and I am grateful.

Every cancer experience is unique, but as this book will show you, some of the moments along the way are universal. By way of introduction to me—the person hoping to gain your trust and guide you through this mess—here's the concise tour of my treatment: I was diagnosed with inflammatory breast cancer (IBC) in November 2012. What makes inflammatory different from other types of breast cancer is how the cancer cells move: The malignant cancer cells block the lymph vessels in the skin, causing redness and swelling in the breast. A rare cancer that spreads rapidly, IBC is diagnosed in approximately 5,000 women in the United States every year. For those who like details, my cancer was ER-positive, PR-positive, and HER2-negative, and I was found to carry a mutated BRCA2 gene. I began chemotherapy within two weeks of diagnosis. When three rounds of Adriamycin/Cytoxan failed, I was told that a clinical drug trial was my only hope. I got into a Phase II clinical trial after being rejected five times. I was finally accepted into a non-randomized, non-placebo-controlled trial for a PARP inhibitor drug called veliparib (made by AbbVie, a spin-off of Abbott Laboratories) at the City of Hope National Medical Center in Duarte, California. To participate in the trial I was required to travel from Northern California to Southern California every week for six months to receive chemotherapy treatment and the accompanying scans and blood work. I had to leave my two young children with my husband, my mom, a babysitter, or my sister for anywhere from one to three days depending on the week. It was torture, mentally and physically.

When my counts were good, some visits ended with just a blood test and then a return trip to the airport, but other visits ended with a round of chemotherapy (Gemzar or carboplatin or both). I had to keep a trial-drug diary listing the dosage, time, and any side effects, as well as follow strict dietary and lifestyle guidelines. The financial and emotional toll was high; there was no insurance or financial coverage for the travel, only the treatment itself. Family, friends, and complete strangers donated air miles, rental car points, hotel rooms, and their time to travel with me. The treatment ended up working—it shrunk the tumor and qualified me for a non-skin-sparing double mastectomy, prophylactic salpingo-oophorectomy (removal of the ovaries and fallopian tubes), and removal of nineteen lymph nodes. That was followed by almost three months of intensive radiation therapy and then breast reconstruction one year later.

My surgery in August 2013 had "clear margins," which means the surgeon got all the detectable cancer surgically. (Cancer cells were described to me by one surgeon as "stars"; the surgeon's job is to remove the stars that have spread out in the targeted area. They get as many of those suckers as possible, but there might be one or two lingering that they can't find.) I have been disease-free since surgery, but I will always be Stage IV because after that number ranking they never "downstage" you; that's your number for life. I still see my oncologist every three months, still get blood work and scans three to four times a year, and will be on hormone therapy for the rest of my life. After about two years on the trial chemo drug, my oncologist took me off it (it had done its job, and the doctor feared that long-term use could cause another secondary type of cancer).

With that one phone call from Dr. Kelley in November 2012, I suddenly entered a world that I had always studiously ignored: the medical world. I hate to have my teeth cleaned, much less sit in paper gowns in waiting rooms and bare all. I used to be so terrified of doctors that I'd break into hives across my chest, causing the doctors to immediately test for allergies. I didn't feel like myself for a couple of months before I went to my GP (general practitioner); I blamed it on being a tired mom. I felt pain in the left side of my chest and noticed some changes in my left breast, and after a round of antibiotics was ineffective, my doctor referred me to a breast surgeon. At no point did I think it could be cancer; everyone kept saying, "Cancer doesn't hurt." I barely got to the breast surgeon for a diagnosis; I tried to put off the appointment so I could help cook that year's Thanksgiving dinner. Dr. Kelley called me the morning after Thanksgiving at 7:00 AM to deliver the news. She told me she didn't like to do it over the phone, but she was in Georgia, and could I please sit down.

Within one hour of that phone call my husband and I were driving to the hospital so I could be admitted for tests and immediate treatment. I was so sick so quickly that much of it occurred in a blur.

Before I was diagnosed, I didn't even know there were types of breast cancer, or even grades of cancer. I was completely, blissfully oblivious to the world of cancer other than the snippets I had heard, read, or seen on television. I started taking notes in a journal on my laptop, writing down my fears and frustrations when I could (especially during the wicked bouts of insomnia created by chemotherapy), and my sister and husband took detailed notes at every appointment. But what I craved (besides icy cold lemonade) was honesty. There are a lot of whispers and pained looks that surround a cancer diagnosis. And there is a lot of silence.

In those first months, I talked to nurses and doctors and X-ray technicians and survivors, but what I didn't hear was anything particularly helpful regarding the day-to-day stuff.

I wanted to hear—or to read—what was really going to happen. What will it feel like to get a needle stuck in my armpit? What will I say to my kids when they ask what happened to my hair? What could I eat? What would chemo feel like? What would radiation do to my skin? What would I look like without breasts? I love nothing more than a plan and a list, and neither was in sight.

I remember so clearly sitting on an exam room table speaking to a radiation oncologist at the MD Anderson Cancer Center in Houston—we were there to get a second opinion—and she looked at me and said, "This fucking sucks. It's okay to cry and say it. Forget the pink warriors. You have cancer and it sucks."

And that was what I craved—to hear someone say something honest about what was happening. I felt so alone, and so isolated, and the only thing I wanted was answers. Books had come to my aid during pregnancy, before job interviews, when I needed to learn a language; my whole life I turned to books for answers. Why not this? The best I could find during the initial steps of my diagnosis were somber hospital brochures titled "Coping with Cancer," filled with photos of half-smiling patients and their caregivers drinking tea.

I needed something else, something honest and at times funny; something real and usable but also a companion, a friendly voice in your ear on a bad day; something that points out the absurdity of your "new normal"; something that addresses the grim specifics that everyone else seems to gloss over; something to flip through when you're wondering "what to expect" from doctors, family, friends.

When I was first diagnosed with cancer, I pictured the Hollywood version of my sick self: a scarf on my head, a blanket on my lap, and an IV in my arm, with one doctor and a few nurses hovering and a family that supported me and cheered me up. Basically me, but bald and slightly nauseous.

It's not like that.

It's a team of doctors, endless nurses, endless scans and blood draws and procedures and confusion and frustration and exhaustion. And that's just the first month.

Now I know that life will never be the same again after a cancer diagnosis. I know you will wish, hope, pray for things to reset and go back to "normal," but they won't. I know now that cancer changes everything.

Oh, how I wish someone had told me that on day one. How I wish someone had given me a book that said it all, in honest/grave/mordantly funny language, and saved me a lot of time and whiplash.

I wish someone had written this book.

My family and I had to educate ourselves while fighting for my life. I didn't have the time or energy for support groups (many of us don't). The research my family and friends did, together with real intel, bits of advice, and vignettes from young survivors, is what *This Is Cancer* is about.

This is everything I have to share on the subject; what I heard and liked, what got me through the appointments, the assaults on my body, and the general shittiness that is being a cancer patient. I want to help you get through this, the most surreal, infuriating journey you'll ever be on. And honestly, I can't stand the word *journey*—I prefer the term *road trip*.

(Imagine a cross-country trip in a covered wagon, in the dead of winter, with an old mule pulling the wagon mile by excruciating mile . . . while cars whiz by.)

Still, this isn't a memoir or a pink ribbon "go, fight, win" book. It's something you can stick in your purse or bag and pull out while you're waiting, and waiting, and waiting in the infinite number of waiting rooms that are in your future. You don't have to read it cover to cover, or even finish the entire thing. It's the one book you should be able to laugh with and feel relieved—*relieved*—to read. To feel "me, too." To feel heard, when no one else in the whole entire world can possibly know what it's like to be you right now.

Now, three-plus years in, and armed with more than my fair share of cancer experience and the stories of others, I have put together this book for first-timers that they desperately need, that I desperately needed.

A book that says things like:

- Chemo will be like the flu times a thousand and will leave a lingering chemical taste in your mouth for months.

- Your children might not look at you when your hair falls out.

- There is no limit to what you will put yourself through when told it might save your life.

- Stay away from the Internet. And don't let anyone tell you "what they looked up" about your diagnosis.

- You'll be surrounded by people but you'll feel lonely, and alone, sometimes.

- Lexapro is Tylenol for the soul.

- You won't be able to manage your life without an entire community helping out, and this will go on for much longer than you think.

- Always question, always persevere.

Said another way, *This Is Cancer* is a chronologically ordered primer, a "what to expect when you're expecting" reference book for the diagnosis you don't want but are stuck with. This is the book that you and your loved ones or support system keep in your "heading to the hospital bag," because it tells you what's going on and keeps you company. Fasten your seat belt and let's get to it.

PART 1

DIAGNOSIS

CHAPTER 1

WELCOME TO CANCERLAND

You will remember the moment of your diagnosis like some people remember where they were on 9/11, or when President Kennedy was shot. You will remember every detail, with great clarity. I don't think it ever goes away. Who tells you, and who designs the road map, kicks off this chapter: the doctors. Think of it as getting into the car before a cross-country drive with a total stranger: You're not sure what music he likes, she might get carsick; he wants to drive all night without stopping, or she wants to stop every hour. Your life is somewhat in your doctors' hands, so it's good to know a few things about their role before it all begins. You can't fully know all of their quirks until you hit the open road, but I'm going to make sure you know how to suss out as many as possible.

The other elements in this new world you've entered are also explained here: nurses, medical centers, paperwork, waiting rooms. And finally, how to pay for it. Because this road trip isn't free, and it's better if you can plan for the bills now that will start filling the mailbox later.

MY DOCTOR IS GOD,
MY DOCTOR IS MORTAL

Let me start by saying I've always been intimidated by doctors. I was always nervous and uneasy sitting on that paper-wrapped exam table. Add the word *oncology* and a few PhDs to that scenario and you've got what I call Doctor Nervous Syndrome. Signs of this syndrome include not telling your doctor every single symptom, not questioning their instructions, and worrying more about their time than yours. I never thought I was allowed to not like my doctor, or question their treatment, or be offended by their behavior. I felt like I was assigned this person and they seemed smart and people respected them so let's get this show on the road.

It was only as things started going wrong in my treatment (read: the tumor wasn't responding as expected) that I discovered I could in fact speak up, that my time (particularly given my diagnosis) was precious, and if anyone should be uncomfortable it should be *them* worried about *me*. I suffered from DNS for many years but was cured a short time after my cancer diagnosis. What helped me get over it was the increased familiarity with my surroundings, getting the lay of the land, and accepting that I was in this situation and would be for a while.

I also came to realize that oncologists in general are not huggy types, that even with a serious diagnosis they don't get too personal, and that they won't necessarily want to hear about your kids. I wanted a cheerleader and a fighter in my oncologist, and eventually I found one, but it took a few tries. This is essential for your treatment, not only physically but mentally as well; they don't need to be your best friend, but they should exhibit some emotion and confidence that sits well with you. You need to trust your doctor and feel comfortable with them, and, ultimately, feel safe with them. If that isn't the case, look for a new provider; there isn't time to waste.

Allowing your doctor to be a human is hard unless you've been raised in a medical family, which I think changes the dynamic and comfort level. There are doctors who will give you their cell phone numbers and actually encourage you to use them, and those you'll speak to only through the switchboard or their nurse (one doctor even told me she wouldn't be available one weekend in case I had any side effects from chemotherapy because she'd "be on the mountain, skiing with the kids").

When and if you get to interview a doctor, consider these details: their bedside manner and their staff's attitude (nursing staff and front desk staff). You're going to be there a lot, so if they're acting like they're doing you a favor, move on to the next doctor. Also weigh whether they are a specialist or researcher. Specialists have more knowledge about a particular cancer than a general oncologist. Researchers are even more familiar with things like new treatments and drug therapies, but they might have limited hours (they spend more time in the research lab and have less availability for seeing patients).

Specialists are not like other doctors—they aren't in the office every day. They usually have surgery or research days and then clinic days, which is when they see patients (they can also run late on clinic days if they're checking on a surgical patient or if they're across town at their research lab). Ask your doctor which days they are available for patients. Also, if you're being treated at a larger medical facility, you will make all your appointments through a scheduler. He or she will coordinate the different appointments with your oncologist and can also sometimes help coordinate appointments in various departments so you can fit as much as possible in one visit.

If your preferred doctor's practice is full and they can't accommodate you, first, ask for referrals. Second, keep trying. I knew one patient who was told that her preferred doctor's practice was full. But she called the office so often that the oncologist relented and offered to consult via video conference. This is also where word of mouth comes in: Email everyone you know, work with, go to the gym or to church with, to see if anyone knows anyone who can help you get an appointment. (For more on word of mouth and second opinions, see page 34.)

When you show up for your appointments, don't be shy. Ask the doctor(s) to explain anything you don't understand. You have to participate in this road trip. (You may not be driving, but you can call out from the backseat.) It may sound simplistic, but asking questions is often the best way to get over your own DNS. Often a doctor either gives a general statement ("You'll feel sick after this round of chemo") or an insanely complicated medical explanation ("Decrease in the lytic component of the left anterior fourth rib adjacent to the costochondral junction"). If you don't understand or you don't have enough information, ask!

Let's finish by discarding the term "doctor's visit." You are no longer visiting; you are officially a citizen of Cancerland.

BEST CANCER HOSPITALS
IN THE UNITED STATES

"Best cancer hospital" is a loaded term. Do you have lung cancer? Colon cancer? Paranasal sinus cancer? The "best" hospital for you is the one that is most familiar with your particular type of cancer. Getting human recommendations, from both doctors and patients (rather than taking advice from the Internet), is the first best step. If you are a researcher by nature, you can check the annual U.S. News & World Report's "Best Hospitals for Cancer" list, on their website. (It's not a fail-safe go-to but rather another piece of research.)

Besides a hospital's reputation, other factors to consider are the geographic location (can you get there easily, or would you need to uproot your family and relocate?) and the size (often a large medical center can coordinate treatment with a smaller hospital that's closer to you). A "high-volume" medical center will most likely have more advanced treatment options than a center who only sees one or two cases a month. Also, consider the support services that are available during and after treatment: Some medical centers offer patient centers with alternative therapies and social services in the same location. These are all questions to ask.

LANGUAGE BARRIERS

When you or your loved one is dealing with cancer, you have to learn a whole new medical language, but if you already speak a language other than English, it can be twice as challenging. Don't hesitate to request translation or interpretative assistance (*interpretative assistance* refers to verbal assistance, while *translation* refers to written materials). This wouldn't be a surprise; at least 350 different languages are currently spoken in U.S. homes, according to a 2015 U.S. Census Bureau report. Hospitals, medical centers, and HMOs often have their own language services, but you might have to contact your city or county to locate language assistance. (Both federal and state law requires that access to a medical interpreter be provided for all patients.)

As with most things in Cancerland, the sooner the better: Tell the scheduler on the phone when making your appointments that you need interpretive or translation services; tell the front desk staff, the nursing staff, and the doctor(s). The medical world refers to patients who need language assistance as LEP—limited English proficiency—and it's added to your medical chart.

The translators are often referred to as medical interpreters or medical linguists. (Sometimes the hospital uses freelancers, which need to be scheduled in advance.) It's crucial that you have a solid understanding of the medical issues, particularly related to prescription medication. Language is a well-documented barrier to health care in the United States, according to the *New England Journal of Medicine*. Some states have strict guidelines for certifying medical interpreters, but it varies by state.

NURSES: THE GOOD, THE BAD, AND EVERYTHING IN BETWEEN

Oh, nurses, I love you dearly and yet sometimes you frustrate me. You soothe, you medicate, you advise, but sometimes you can be mean and moody. Often it feels like dealing with a three-year-old; sometimes the nurses are all smiles and sometimes they might as well scream, "You're not the boss of me." In general, nurses are amazing, supportive caregivers. Still, paving the road is a good thing; smiling first is never a bad idea.

You will meet many different kinds of nurses on this road trip, including oncology nurses, nurse practitioners, advanced practice nurses, registered nurses, nurses' assistants, clinical nurse specialists, nurse anesthetists, nurse navigators, nurse case managers, licensed practical nurses, and surgical nurses. They all have a different vibe, and you'll get to know the nuances; nurses in the ER are completely different from the clinical nurses who run drug trials, and the oncology nurses could not be more different from the recovery room post-op nurses in the hospital. They take care of so many details: explaining certain procedures, calling in prescriptions, checking surgical scars, and generally acting as a go-between for you and the doctor. Remember, the nurses are all there to support the team, which includes you, and they usually have more time than the doctors to go over quality-of-life issues. Talk to them and ask away; they usually have insight and knowledge that is hard to find elsewhere.

As I hit bumps in the road—bump after bump—there were nurses who understood when I needed to get a quick answer to a question, or needed a sympathetic ear, a little bit of encouragement, or a distraction. The radiation oncology nurse was so kind and thoughtful when I showed her the rash that had developed that I thought she was going to cry. (She also returned my calls without delay, even on her days off.) The "plastics" nurse always chatted me up as she was injecting saline into my breast expanders, trying to distract me from the syringe being plunged into what was formerly my nipple. The oncology nurse at City of Hope gave me a huge smile and a hug on my final infusion day, high-fiving me as I walked out of the room.

I suggest bringing gifts of food to the nurse's station: cookies or pizza, or bins of popcorn or pretzels, especially if you're staying over in the hospital. As with everything in life, being rude gets you nowhere. It's the nurses who administer medication, but be ready to argue if you still feel pain, especially in the middle of the night in the hospital. Be aware that if there are any issues about medications, the nurse must contact the doctor to clarify or get clearance, and they might not want to call the doctor in the middle of the night. Hospitals are not always models of continuity, so when the shift changes you might have to start all over with explanations and describing your symptoms to the next nurse. Just be ready to repeat yourself.

PAPERWORK:
PASSPORT FOR CANCER PATIENTS

Bring a pen. That is my number one piece of advice when you're heading to the doctor's office or medical center. Even though medical records are moving to electronic format, you will still have to fill out hundreds of pages of documents once you're diagnosed. It's paperwork: some long, some short, some financial, most of it medical history. If your health insurance is through a health maintenance organization (HMO) such as Kaiser Permanente, you will most likely only have to fill out forms once since the medical information is typically integrated.

Pen and paper (and computers) are as much a part of cancer as blood tests. The endless forms will make your head spin. Patient forms, liability waivers, and clipboards are the norm. I tried to read every line of every piece of paper, which was sometimes alarming. But I wasn't always in the best state of mind. Be sure you have someone with you to go over the forms.

To keep it all straight, it helps to make a cheat sheet with answers to the most common questions: what medications you've been on, both prescription and over-the-counter; any allergies; any adverse reactions; symptoms; for women, date of last menstrual period; family history of major illnesses like strokes or diabetes; names and contact information of other physicians you've seen. (You can also include details such as your blood type and your normal blood pressure.) You will be handed clipboards with papers again and again, and you will swear you already filled this one out, but it's useless to protest. Just consult your cheat sheet, fill it out, and hand it to the front desk.

The most intimidating paperwork moment for me occurred when I started my clinical trial at City of Hope. A staff member walked me and my family into a room that looked like it belonged in a bank: dark wood paneling, plush rugs, a perfectly green potted plant in the corner, a leather blotter on the desk. And then the paperwork began, this time pages and pages and pages to be signed with a big black pen. (If you're entering a clinical drug trial, there is even more paperwork with all kinds of scary fine print.) If I hadn't known any better I would have thought I had just taken out a mortgage (which I kind of did, in the form of tiny green chemotherapy pills). I was thrilled to be there for treatment, but this was a surreal experience.

There is also paperwork that you must carry around and present at each medical appointment. Three must-haves for your patient visits: your medical record card (most larger hospitals and medical centers issue them to patients at the first appointment), your health insurance card (if applicable), and your driver's license or state identification card.

WAITING ROOMS: THE HOLDING TANKS

Waiting rooms will be your new neighborhood, your new coffee shop. Wherever you hung out the most before you got sick, the time you used to spend there will now be spent in doctor's offices and hospital waiting rooms.

There are two levels of waiting rooms: the outer waiting room and then the inner exam room. The outer room is like an airport waiting area, and the inner is the sanctum, onboard the plane. The thing about the second room is it's not exactly freedom—you're not in the air yet. Once you're in, you're one step closer. But then you're just waiting in a cloth or paper gown. You will wait; it's not a matter of if, it's a matter of how long. My worst day of waiting was close to three hours in the inner exam room. (My father raised me to take reading materials—books, magazines, newspapers—wherever I go, and that has gotten me through a lot of waiting.) Make sure to bring your own; the magazine selection is usually better in the second room, but there are no guarantees.

There are also two sub-levels of waiting rooms: waiting to see the doctor and waiting for a procedure or an infusion. The shortest waiting time I ever had was for radiation, and that's fairly common; patients are seen at exact times because the setup of the machine takes so much time and precision. (For more on radiation therapy, see Radiation 101 in chapter 4.)

Part of the general bureaucracy of the medical community is the wait time for each particular doctor: some are notoriously late and some are notoriously on time. At my oncologist's office there is a large white board that lists every doctor and the average wait time. I love this; at least you can grab a coffee or walk around the block instead of sitting in the room getting irritated. (The front desk might even be convinced to take your cell phone number and call you when the doctor is almost ready to see you.)

The remarkable thing to me about waiting rooms is the wide array of entertainment. Some have flat-screen TVs and fresh magazines from the actual current year, and some even have Wi-Fi. Others have ragged ten-year-old magazines and prison-like TVs bolted to the wall, and no sound. Some medical centers have lending libraries, generally full of thrillers and romance novels, where patients and their caregivers can borrow, read, and return books (it's the cancer book swap).

When you walk in the front door, ask the volunteers at the information desk—who are often bursting with information and eager to tell you all about the hospital—about any lending libraries on site.

As for food and drink, some waiting rooms have a water dispenser, coffee, tea, and even juice. Some just have a lone drinking fountain and sad Styrofoam (yes, Styrofoam) cups. Bring a large water bottle just in case. Some have ample chairs—one would think that would be a priority for a facility frequented by sick people—while others have so few it's like everyone is playing musical chairs whenever someone disappears to the bathroom or the cafeteria. People do pack their own food, but beware the patients that bring in the buffet. If your sense of smell is sensitive, pick a chair down the hall. I've seen feasts worthy of a banquet hall in large hospital waiting areas. When you do pack a snack, keep in mind that it should be something that can sit for hours without refrigeration, won't smell awful when opened (like tuna), and is relatively easy to eat in front of people (skip the peas in the pod and peanuts in their shell). There is nothing more irritating than listening to—and watching—someone eat peanuts in their shell when you feel as sick as a dog. Don't do that to your fellow patients.

The other element of the waiting room is listening for your name to be called. It's like a twisted game show: When the door opens and a nurse appears, everyone kind of tenses and leans forward to hear their name called. Sometimes you wait so long you'll answer to anything. "Barbara Long?" the nurse calls, and you, Jane Smith, almost shout, "Yes, yes, that's me!" They give you about three shouts before they move on to the next patient, making the experience akin to flying standby. The adrenaline is flowing and you're darting your eyes around, sizing up the competition. It's the strangest feeling, because logic tells you that you're all there for the same reason and the doctor has to see everyone eventually. But somehow the pressure of that twenty-minute differential takes over, especially when you're having a bad day. For me, that meant I could get outside twenty minutes earlier and do something remotely more fun than being poked and prodded. Or get to the airport for an earlier flight home.

There's also a certain hierarchy to the waiting room. There are character types that exist no matter where you're being treated. There's always the sickest, longest-reigning patient who loves to talk about their medical condition and one-up you (I call them either The Queen Bee or The King); one with a cluster of relatives that take up half the chairs; one sleeping patient, often snoring; one glued to his or her cell phone; one watching an iPad at top volume without headphones; and one watching the television like it's God himself, even if the sound is off.

CANCERSPEAK, PART 1: A TRANSLATION GUIDE

They speak a different language in Cancerland. Here are some basic terms and phrases you will hear repeatedly in the oncology world during your road trip, and what they really mean. Think of it as a translation guide.

DOCTOR: "I'm concerned."
MEANING: He/she is very concerned, borderline terrified.

NURSING STAFF: "The doctor will be with you shortly."
MEANING: The doctor will be with you in two to three hours.

DOCTOR: "This medication should help with the discomfort."
MEANING: "You can try this first, but we both know you'll
be calling me tomorrow because it either won't work or it
will make you throw up."

PATIENT: "This medication isn't working."
DOCTOR: "It should be."
MEANING: "You're sure you're taking the right dosage?"

DOCTOR: "I'll need to see you for a follow-up in three weeks."
MEANING: "Start calling my scheduler this instant and pray
that in three weeks you'll be able to make it for a 7:46 AM
appointment, which really means 10:45 AM, and then we
still might have inconclusive results."

DOCTOR: "You might feel some discomfort."
MEANING: This will hurt like hell.

DOCTOR: "I'll need you to fast for that blood work."
MEANING: No form of water or food shall pass your lips for
twelve hours prior to the needle being stuck in your arm,
so you'll need to stay away from the kitchen or sit in the
car with your eyes closed and try not to imagine a buttery
croissant.

BLOOD TECHNICIAN: "I can't find the order in the system."
MEANING: "I have to call the resident, who will call someone

else, and on and on, and it will take thirty minutes to reach anyone who knows anything, so settle in with a magazine."

ONCOLOGIST: "We need to get you into a trial."
MEANING: Your regular chemo protocol or regimen isn't working. You need to make sure that they find you a non-randomized, non-placebo controlled drug trial in the United States. This means you know you are receiving the actual drug (not a placebo). Also, you're running out of time. (This is what happened to me, but other patients seek trials to prevent recurrence or myriad other reasons.)

DOCTOR: "The tests came back negative."
MEANING: This is a positive thing, as in, good news. (You want to be positive in your attitude and negative in your tests, I discovered.)

THE COST OF CANCER (LITERALLY): MEDICAL BILLS, FEES, AND FINANCES

Having cancer is expensive. There's no other way to say it. Hopefully you have health insurance, which can defray the costs significantly, or you have money saved up. If not, don't despair; there are ways to find help, so don't let financial worries derail your focus on treatment. Cancer treatment involves hundreds of office visits (and often hospital stays), laboratory tests, and other medical tests, which leads to thousands (or hundreds of thousands, or even millions) of dollars in medical bills. Whether it's insurance co-payments or medical center bills, it all has to be paid. The

American Cancer Society cites an Agency for Healthcare Research and Quality (AHRQ) study that found overall expenditures for cancer treatment in 2011 were $88.7 billion. Half that cost was for outpatient and doctor visits, 35 percent was inpatient hospital costs, and 11 percent was for prescription medications.

If You Have Health Insurance

Health insurance is an insanely complicated subject that I can't do justice to here. But here are some basics. Medical treatment is paid in one of two ways: (1) through your health insurance company, where you pay the premiums, co-pays, and any deductible, and the company reimburses the provider (the doctor, hospital, laboratory, or other provider); or (2) you pay the doctor or hospital directly, then get reimbursed by the insurance company. An HMO is treated like a health insurance model: You pay a monthly premium and maybe a deductible, depending on the plan you've purchased.

Few people read the fine print when they buy health insurance, but you need to be on top of every detail of your policy. If you're not up for handling the details and talking to the insurance company, sign your insurance company's medical disclosure waiver so your partner, spouse, family member, or other designated person can talk about your case on your behalf.

If you, the patient, have to pay up front and deal with the bills yourself, I strongly suggest finding a family member or friend who can help you. You simply won't have the energy to manage the bills that will arrive almost weekly from the insurance company and the hospitals and the laboratories. (The paperwork I found particularly amusing was the notices from the insurance company that said in bold letters, "This is not a bill." All it meant was that a bill was coming.) Keeping track of all this paperwork requires concentration and organizational skills, neither of which you will have in the throes of chemotherapy, or radiation, or after surgery. A well-organized set of folders on your computer—or even three-ring binders or expandable file folders—will be key to keeping things organized. Keep folders for medical information and a record of tests, procedures, and office visits, as well as folders for bills and insurance records. Match the financial binder with your medical binder, where you keep your own set of CDs containing your scans, office visit summaries, and lab results that the medical center gives you.

You can, and should, request that the insurance company assign you a "concierge," case worker, or case manager who can help manage your case, meaning the bills and co-pays and forms—the mountain of paperwork that is about to be generated. It's comforting to have the name and number (or email) of an actual person you can turn to with questions or when you face a roadblock from a doctor or hospital.

Keep in mind that some medical practices and medical centers will require proof of insurance before they'll see you, and if you have not cleared the prior authorizations they will expect payment the day of the appointment. That is why it's crucial to know exactly what your coverage includes and the co-payments, referrals, and authorizations that will be necessary.

Your Health Insurance Policy: The Fine Print

These are the details of your health insurance policy that you need to find out immediately after you're diagnosed (call the customer service number on the back of your insurance card for the quickest way to get answers):

- Are there pre-authorizations or prior authorizations required for any procedures or treatments prescribed by your doctor(s)? If treatment is denied, you need to be ready to gather more information in order to appeal (and preferably have your doctor get involved).

- If you have a fee-for-service plan (a.k.a. an indemnity plan), what is the yearly deductible and what is the co-pay percentage?

- Are second (and third, if needed) medical opinions covered? (See page 34 for more on second opinions.)

- If you're considering participating in a clinical trial, what kind of follow-up care will be covered under your plan? (For more on clinical trials, see chapter 4.)

There are also federal laws that require health insurance companies to pay for specific procedures. For example, the Women's Health and Cancer Rights Act (WHCRA), passed in 1998, requires group health plans and health insurance companies that offer mastectomy coverage to pay for reconstructive surgery after mastectomy. (This does not apply to Medicaid and Medicare recipients, however.) For more on reconstructive surgery after mastectomy, see Breast Reconstruction in chapter 4.

You can get detailed information about WHCRA from the Department of Labor (DOL) Employee Benefits Security Administration website (http://www.dol.gov/ebsa/publications/whcra.html).

If You Don't Have Health Insurance

If you don't have health insurance, you are among 41 million uninsured Americans (a US Census statistic from 2014). The Affordable Care Act (ACA), passed in 2010, requires that every American be deemed eligible for health insurance, regardless of preconditions or other factors; go to the HHS website for complete details. The American Cancer Society also has detailed information for patients about how the ACA affects cancer patients and their families (www.cancer.org/acs/groups/content/@editorial/documents/document/acspc-026864.pdf).

Needless to say, your first question to the doctor who is offering a possibly lifesaving drug isn't "What does it cost?" but rather "How can I get it?" It could be a pill, or a prescription, or an office visit. But the costs do add up quickly (be prepared to pay not only the cost of the drug but a facility fee, doctor fee, and drug administration fee). And the bills continue even after you are sent home cancer-free: follow-up visits and tests can go on for at least six months after your last treatment and may last for years.

But even if you're facing what can seem like huge, insane, and overwhelming medical bills, know that there are many, many organizations out there—nonprofits, foundations, and others—that can help patients prepare, deal with, and sometimes pay for, cancer treatment. Some help patients write a financial plan; some help with cancer treatment-related costs such as travel or childcare; and some will help pay for treatment directly. Some medical centers have endowments specifically set up to assist patients in need. (See the Resources section for more specific information.) It's just like college financial aid and scholarships: It's out there—you just have to know how to go after it.

Some medical centers have social work services or licensed social workers that can work with you for a reduced or no cost (and some can even help you by phone if you are too sick to come to the office or if you live far away from the medical center). These services can help with things like:

- Applying for short- or long-term disability
- Understanding your health insurance policy
- Finding other grant money and local programs that you might qualify for

Many foundations and programs fund patients on a local level, making it impossible to list them all here. For example, the Firefly Sisterhood (www.fireflysisterhood.org) is a non-profit that helps breast cancer patients who live in Minnesota. In Washington, DC, the Whitman-Walker Health Center's Mautner Project provides direct services to members of the LGBT community who have been diagnosed with cancer, including transportation to treatments, patient navigation, and other assistance. Call them at (202) 745-7000 for more information. (See Resources for more programs like this.)

The Hidden Cost of Cancer

Besides medical costs, there are hundreds of random (and often unexpected) fees and costs that come with being a cancer patient. And there are many nonprofits that can help with these specific costs; see the Resources section for more specifics.

Here's the short list of fees and costs to help you prepare:

- Parking fees. Parking can become a major cost. Ask your doctor if you qualify for a temporary disabled parking placard, which can get you free or reduced parking fees. It's a fairly simple procedure: The doctor fills out a form; you go to your local DMV with the paperwork and receive the placard. Display it on your rearview mirror; it's generally valid for six months. It can make all the difference if you have to walk only one block instead of ten; when you are tired and sore from radiation, every ten feet counts. Your new placard might also qualify you for free or discounted parking in hospital lots, city lots, or airports; be sure to ask the parking attendant.

- Taxis, car service, tolls, or public transportation.

- Gas costs, particularly if you are driving great distances to treatment.

- Costs of over-the-counter medications, including creams and bandages.

- Pharmacy delivery fees if you need to have medication delivered.

- Food and beverage costs at the hospital (particularly if you're traveling for treatment).

- Any fees required to obtain medical records.

- Medical "accessories" like lymphedema sleeves or compression stockings. These are often available over the counter and then reimbursed by your health insurance company. But the up-front costs can be high: For example, a set of lymphedema sleeves cost around $200. Be sure to ask your doctor for a prescription for these items.

- Cost of wigs, hats, and scarves if you are undergoing chemotherapy.

- Childcare costs.

- Physical therapy, which insurance will often not cover completely.

- Psychotherapy or mental health costs, also often not completely covered by insurance.

- Any alternative therapies you might be trying to help minimize side effects of treatment, such as chiropractic care, acupuncture, or hypnosis.

- Any clothing you may need to accommodate treatment or recovery, such as button-front tops, elastic-waist pants, or new shoes if your feet swell.

- Food costs at home. If you're not receiving meals from friends and you don't feel like cooking, you will most likely eat take-out food. Also, if your treatment affects your mouth or your ability to swallow and you can only consume liquids, you will need a food processor or blender to puree foods.

If you use credit cards for cancer-related expenses it's easy to run up debt. If you need credit counseling, contact the National Foundation for Credit Counseling (www.njcc .org). They provide free, confidential advice about managing credit card bills and payments. See Resources for more information about organizations that can provide credit counseling or financial assistance.

FIRST OPINION

Not everyone seeks more than one medical opinion when they receive a cancer diagnosis. Whether you choose to or not, know that it is your decision. This is not the time to worry about hurting anyone's feelings or to enter into medical center politics. It's your body and your right to talk to as many doctors as you want. That said, this is what usually happens after you get your first opinion or diagnosis: The oncologist generally meets with her or his colleagues in a weekly meeting called a Tumor Board. (I originally thought patients were invited and possibly refreshments were served; they are not and no.) Most oncology groups have four or five specialists that focus on a particular type of cancer, including an oncology surgeon and a radiation oncologist. The doctors discuss the case and treatment and come to a conclusion about a treatment plan.

Then the oncologist assigned to your case meets with you in an exam room to deliver the news. They go over test results and present the treatment plan. Bring someone with you (husband/wife/partner/family member) to hold your hand and take notes. Write down everything they say, even if the doctor says he or she will write it for you. Written notes are crucial, particularly when you're piecing everything together in the very beginning.

The oncologist will generally focus on immediate treatment; for example, if you need chemotherapy, surgery, and radiation, she'll tell you in detail about the chemotherapy plan and then send you to the surgeon's office and the radiation oncologist's office to meet them and discuss their specific plans. If surgery won't happen immediately, the surgeon will give you brief details and then schedule a more detailed meeting as your treatment progresses and a surgery date is actually scheduled. (I talked briefly to a surgeon upon diagnosis, and the thought of surgery scared me more than anything. And then I had to think about it for eight more months.)

I highly suggest you avoid the Internet at this point; I can't say this enough. Going online to research anything about your condition can only end in tears, unless you happen to have a medical background, are married to a professor of medicine, or have access to a medical library. And even then, I wouldn't advise it. You can come up with all sorts of ideas that lead to scary places. (The same goes for any friends trying to "help" by looking up your diagnosis.) Yes, knowledge is power. But you must educate yourself from reputable sources only. That is the only reason I'm alive today, my sister reminds me constantly. We had no idea about the options available, but my family found knowledgeable people who pushed and pushed until we found something that offered a chance at survival.

SECOND OPINION

If you decide you do need to either confirm a diagnosis or get another option for treatment, you can opt for a second opinion. This is particularly true if you have a type of cancer that is unusual or aggressive, and if your health insurance covers it. Insurance companies are all over the map on the topic, though: HMOs, for example, usually don't pay for patients to seek opinions outside the HMO, while other insurance companies require a second opinion before treatment can begin. Remember, you always have the time for a second opinion. This is *your* illness, and you still have a say in what is happening to you. Whether to get one or not is a matter of personal preference, but if finances or geography are the only things preventing you from seeking out another option, find a way to make it happen. There are so many resources and foundations that can help with the cost; even crowd-funding has become an option for individuals to raise money for medical costs. (See Resources for organizations that can help fund the cost of getting a second opinion, including any travel that may be necessary.)

Before you seek a medical center or doctor for a second opinion, do some research. The most critical research my family did was to ask around about the reputation of the various medical centers and doctors; it becomes clear fairly quickly who the respected hospitals and doctors are in a particular field. If there's a doctor that is well-known in the field, try and get in touch with them. Call, email, fax—whatever you can do to fight for contact. The worst thing that can happen is they say no.

Just be aware that your primary physician or oncologist might not be thrilled by the news that you're seeking another opinion. This shocked me, particularly because I was literally fighting for my life. I remember very clearly watching my sister and husband on the phone trying to get medical records from my oncologist's office, and they put up resistance, as though we were asking them to do us a favor. And when I got on the phone myself, it was still a struggle. It was unbelievable, and distressing, and not a good way to begin the "road trip."

And be ready: Getting a second opinion requires getting an entirely new set of scans, blood work, and everything else—basically starting over at another medical center. You will need all of the original test results and your medical record as well. Make a list of questions before the appointment, including asking the doctor to verify the original pathology and diagnosis and explain any differences in treatment approach.

And be aware that the second opinion might be the same as the first. But that's the risk (and the benefit). Differences among medical centers can be significant, both in research and faculty. This is normal; how one medical center approaches a surgery might be entirely different from another center with a new surgeon who has learned a cutting-edge technique. And geography plays a part: A smaller rural hospital might not have access to the machines and equipment that a larger urban facility does. This is particularly true with radiation therapy. For example, right after I was diagnosed it was the standard procedure at one facility to tattoo patients with a small dot to mark the area for later treatment, but doctors at another medical center told me they "don't do that anymore."

A third opinion is also an option. Again, if you have a rare type of cancer or diagnosis, a third opinion is commonplace. You will need yet another set of records and scans to bring with you, but you will also have to complete another round of tests and scans at the third medical institution.

To me, the hardest part about hearing multiple opinions were the moments when the doctors disagreed. I had family members with me at all the meetings and appointments, and they took notes for me. But deciding which opinion to listen to was an overwhelming situation, to put it mildly. At one point, when faced with two options in two different cities, I asked my oncologist, "If I were your daughter, what would you have me do?" And when he told me his answer, I chose that one.

Another aspect of diagnosis I was completely unprepared for was medical photography—commonly used in specialties like plastic surgery and dermatology. Some large medical centers have medical photographers that photograph the part of your body that has cancer (in my case, my breasts) as part of the initial exam. The breast cancer photos are from the neck down—the goal is to photograph the cancer and not your face—but it was a total surprise to me when a photographer walked into the exam room and asked me to undress. (It was a woman, but still.) I was happy to comply since I knew the photos would benefit other patients and physicians, but it would have been nice to have a heads-up. Be sure you ask how the photos will be used and sign a waiver if you have any qualms about it.

OFF THE CLOCK: WORK AND CANCER

Finding out you have cancer is hard enough, but discovering that the treatment might affect your job can be terrifying. Even the most basic thing like telling your boss can be wildly uncomfortable. This is a huge topic that deserves more space than I can devote here, but here are a few guidelines to get you through the initial shock and help bring a little control to this part of your life so you can focus on you.

First, tell your boss or supervisor. You don't have to go into extreme detail, but be ready to give an outline in a calm voice. If you have a job that isn't very physically demanding, you might be able to continue working. Leave the possibility open until you see how you react to treatment (there are obviously cases where this is impossible, but in general it's something to consider). If you get pushback from your boss or supervisor or have specific concerns relating to your diagnosis and your job, consider consulting an employment attorney (there are legal aid options for cancer patients; see Resources). Cancer in the workplace is covered in the Americans with Disabilities Act (ADA) and the ADA Amendments Act (ADAAA) of 2008 and is overseen by the U.S. Equal Employment Opportunity Commission (EEOC). The ADA applies to employers with fifteen or fewer employees, and the EEOC website has detailed info for both employers and employees (see Resources for more information).

After you've told your boss, ask to meet with someone from your company's Human Resources department. If you work for a large company, they might be able to assign you one person you can work with the entire time. The HR person should go over all of your benefits, including how many sick days and vacation days you've accrued and how much unpaid and other paid time off is available. They should also review your health insurance policy (which you need to then review again yourself with the health insurance company) and your retirement account if you have one through work. Be sure you have all the paperwork set up so that your spouse/partner and your children are included on your life insurance and other benefits. You should also ask about the company's medical leave policy. (For more information on your caregiver's rights to take time off to care for you, see Taking Care of Your Caretaker in chapter 3.)

A few things to remember about the Big C and your job:

- If you belong to a union, contact your representative about what is covered medically as well as job security policies.

- Talking to your coworkers can be tricky. You need to decide what you want to share. Legally, your boss is not allowed to divulge any information, but if you work in a small work environment or you have an obvious physical symptom, it might be unrealistic to expect that coworkers wouldn't observe or hear things.

- Talk to your boss about options like telecommuting. With high-speed Internet and a home computer there might be alternatives to being in the office, even if it's for a short period of time.

- Allow yourself to be angry, sad, or whatever emotion comes up surrounding your job. For many people their job is a huge part of their identity, and leaving it even temporarily because of cancer is an unbelievable blow.

- Be realistic with yourself about your ability to do your job. If your mental or physical state is changing, listen to the people around you. You might refuse to acknowledge changes, and someone close to you might need to give you a nudge into reality. (The week before I was diagnosed I had interviewed for a writing gig, a book that I was really excited to work on. I remember emailing the literary agent, telling her I had gotten some medical news that took me out of the running but I hoped to be back in a few months. Little did I know—or realize—it would be years before I would have the mental and physical capacity to do what I love to do on a professional level.)

Social Security

Social Security benefits aren't just for your grandparents; they might be a financial option for you. Applying is a bit of a process, but you may qualify for benefits if you've been in the workforce for a certain number of years and your illness looks like it will last (or has already lasted) more than one year, or "is expected to end in death" (the SSA's words, not mine). You must fill out an Adult Disability Report, available in the Forms section on the Social Security Administration (SSA) website, and if it's approved you will receive a check from the SSA; the amount depends on how long you worked and how much you earned before your illness. Your spouse and children may be eligible to receive benefits on your behalf as well. If you're unable to fill out the form, the SSA has representatives who can help you. You do not need any medical records other than what you have; with your permission the SSA can request records directly from the doctor.

JOURNALS, EMAILS, BLOGS, AND OTHER PUBLIC AIRINGS

Discussing or sharing your diagnosis is a highly personal choice. I didn't hesitate; I emailed my group of friends within a day or two of finding out. We lived in a small community next to the small town where my sister and her family lived—the town where we grew up. A lot of old friends and acquaintances remained in the community, and I felt comfortable sharing, particularly because we knew so many cancer survivors in town. That doesn't mean there weren't awkward moments in the grocery store or awkward moments in general. But we felt supported by having everyone know what was going on. And in the end, that's what ultimately helped save my life: Someone told someone else who knew a particular doctor at the University of California, San Francisco, who specialized in breast cancer and scheduled an appointment for me.

However, I am very aware that I had a common cancer, something that didn't involve a high level of shame or invite any sort of public shaming. I have heard some survivors of cancers such as lung and tongue—people who never smoked or chewed tobacco or anything else, for what it's worth—discuss how hard it was to talk about their diagnosis because people assumed that they had caused it. And some types of cancers are just more awkward to discuss. Sharing a prostate cancer or colorectal cancer diagnosis that could leave you impotent and incontinent isn't exactly dinner-party conversation. Cultural or religious reasons might also influence someone's decision to keep a diagnosis private. So when people talk about "breaking the news," it's okay to have your own reasons for not sharing.

I privately wrote down everything to preserve the experience and feelings for my kids in case I didn't make it: Thoughts, feelings, bits and pieces of life advice I had always planned to tell them. I wanted them to know what I was thinking and how hard I was working to stay with them. I eventually shared some of my writing with certain friends and family. But let me be clear: Before cancer I was not a person who would write the word *breast* in an email to people I didn't know or use it in a sentence when talking to my parents. The deeper I got into my treatment, the more I started using the word *breast* like a medical professional: as a term that describes a part of the female anatomy. Nothing more, nothing less.

I also wrote about my daily experiences in a journal, sometimes by hand but mostly on my laptop. I've always been a writer, so for me writing is a comfort. I've always been better communicating through writing than in person. It made it easier to tell people what was going on instead of talking about it. And frankly, I was just too tired to talk all the time anyway. If you don't like to write but want to record your experience, make voice recordings with a laptop computer or a voice memo app on a cell phone or tablet. Or ask a friend to transcribe or write down your thoughts.

I also felt that the more I wrote and shared my writing, the more people understood what it was actually like week by week. People are curious and want to know what you're experiencing, but for obvious reasons they don't want to ask too many questions. I wanted to give them this information and explain the "real" cancer experience. I was not into social media at the time, so I used good old-fashioned emails.

However, I did have a friend suggest setting up a community website where people could sign up for tasks like making dinner or dropping off diapers. These websites can also become part of long-distance caregiving, where family or friends who live far away can have items shipped to you or help in other ways like direct financial assistance. Having one website makes coordinating everything so much easier on your caregiver. (It's also useful for sending out notices, such as asking visitors to refrain from wearing perfume or fragrance if you can't tolerate it after treatment.)

There are "care calendar" websites—what I call "helper" websites—that have a section where you can update your community and send out group updates and even post photos. For most of the sites, users have to submit their email addresses and be approved by the designated person to become part of your community, so the information can't be viewed by the general public. (This varies, however, so be sure to read the fine print on the website before creating a page.) These websites include Lotsa Helping Hands and CaringBridge; see Resources for a complete list. Some sites are specifically geared to cancer patients, such as MyLifeLine.org. (Some patients use these and other crowdfunding websites to raise money for treatment; see page 282 for more information.)

Using social media to share and/or discuss your experience is a very personal choice. Some survivors I spoke to feel comforted by online forums and/or social media and see it as a resource or even a solace. (Misery loves company, right?) Others feel overwhelmed (especially if the good wishes are being messaged to you on the hour, every hour, for months at a time). Another thing to consider is the "comedown," the eventual slowdown in the constant communication by friends and even family; if you are facing a long or prolonged treatment, it's inevitable the attention on you will fade. Seeing that happen in real time on a social media outlet might make it a little more unbearable than it already is.

It's also important to remember that what is posted can't easily be undone. This is medical information you are posting; especially if you're a young adult, do you want that information (text and/or photos) on the Internet for eternity? It's something to think about. Do what feels right for you, and don't feel pressured to share (or not share).

FRIENDS TO SURROUND YOURSELF WITH

Friends are key to getting through a cancer diagnosis. Regardless of whether you have family nearby or relatives who can relocate to help you through treatment, chances are it will be your friends who provide the daily support. It's friends who can organize a group to get tasks done and friends who can distract you from the dark moments. While your family grapples with the wide range of emotions around your diagnosis, friends can be the more reliable lifeline to keep actual life happening: getting the kids to school, getting meals on the table, feeding the cat, and arranging rides to treatment.

Of all the times in the world that you need to rely on people—family, friends, or community—*this* is the time. This is when you say "yes" instead of "no." This is the time to trouble people, to bother them, to take them up on their offers. You will need them. Getting help is more complicated if you've chosen not to share your diagnosis with many people, but it can still be done. Your friends want to feel helpful; otherwise they retreat, not knowing what to say or do. They often feel powerless, which might come out in strange ways. Seeing someone who is very sick can trigger their own fears about illness and dying; don't take it personally.

Friends helped me and my family with the smallest things: buying groceries for us while they were already heading to the store or dropping off diapers and baby wipes from Costco. Most importantly, friends were able to help babysit and arrange fun playdates that distracted the kids and left me time to heal and recover.

Requesting a specific task is the best way to have someone help you. For example, my daughter had ballet on Wednesdays, so having a friend pick her up from school and take her to class freed up my family to help with the baby and pick up prescriptions or the other hundreds of things that needed to be done. Often I couldn't be left alone, so we asked friends to rotate being my "person" at home. One friend drove me to medical appointments, while another took the kids for the day so my husband could have some downtime.

The key attributes of a cancer friend are patience, reliability, a sense of humor, the ability not to cry when they look at you, and the ability to cook or at least grocery shop. A friend who can censor herself is an added bonus; you can do without the little comments like, "You'll be fine!" A cancer friend squeezes your hand without a word when they don't know what to say; they show up and sit by you when you are in bed for weeks at a time; they help organize playdates for your kids when you don't have the energy; and they never expect a thank-you. You thank them, of course, but they do all of these things behind the scenes without involving you, which is what you need.

People did things for me—even people I had met maybe once or twice before I got sick—that made all the difference in the world. My friend Carrie drove forty-five minutes in the pouring rain to bring a CD of scans to a doctor to review to help me qualify for a clinical drug trial. My mom was watching my kids, my sister was trying to get other medical records while managing her three kids, and my dad was with me while I was getting a CT scan. Carrie walked in soaking wet with the CD in her hand like an angel from above. Those moments are pure acts of kindness. I was a person who barely wanted someone to rearrange my pantry while I was pregnant, and now I had a community, and virtual strangers, who were decorating my house for Christmas, bringing me meals, driving me to appointments, and helping me put stamps on Christmas cards. It was beyond humbling, and still brings me to my knees with gratitude. Friends of friends sent me scarves, slippers, even ice cream. The old phrase "the kindness of strangers" is suddenly more striking when you get sick.

My mother raised me to send thank-you cards, and God help me if I don't send one within three days of receiving a gift. But this is the time to put them on hold. I sent email updates to my community and said thank you in that way, and then later—sometimes up to a year later—I wrote personal cards. But don't even think about it right now. Again, that energy is better spent on you and your family. (When you are ready for thank-you notes, see the sidebar in chapter 12 for some easy, creative ideas.)

Cancer friends and caregivers:

- Do things without asking.

- Are problem solvers.

- Walk the dog, vacuum the dog hair, feed the cat, or clean the litter box.

- Mow the lawn or take care of the houseplants.

- Change lightbulbs or sweep the kitchen floor.

- Organize the mail/paperwork/bills that tend to pile up when you're just diagnosed.

- Bring a box of pastries from your favorite bakery with them when they drop by.

- Act as screeners. They email, answer the phone, or handle people who want to come by. You, the patient, should not answer the phone unless you're up to it. Say no, say you can't talk, say I'm not up to it. I didn't want to waste my precious time on the phone rehashing things with well-meaning, faraway friends. I sent emails and then read their responses when I felt like it. (If you are what I call a phone person, don't worry; there will be ample time for you to call everyone in the world while you wait at the pharmacy, while someone is driving you to treatment, or when you're sitting on the couch recovering. Just be polite about it if you're in the waiting room or in line at the pharmacy and step outside rather than gabbing away.)

That said, not all friends will be there for you. Prepare yourself for friends who disappear, drop in sporadically, or don't behave the way you expect them to. You've got to deal with what you've got, and sometimes that means letting go of people who you thought would be with you through everything. Later on, when you're through treatment, you can decide whether to circle back to them. But for now, put your focus on where it's needed: you and your family.

For more on friends and how to encourage compassionate behavior, see page 83.

The Pink Ribbon, and the Other Colors of Cancer

The pink ribbon, now the ubiquitous symbol of breast cancer, was introduced in 1991 when pink ribbons were distributed to all participants in the Komen New York City Race for the Cure. The race was part of what was then known as the Susan G. Komen Breast Cancer Foundation (the name was changed in 2007 to Susan G. Komen for the Cure), founded by Nancy G. Brinker, whose sister, Susan, died of breast cancer.

Other cancer causes have adopted the idea and made ribbons in different colors for other cancers; dark blue is for colon cancer, gray is for brain cancer, clear is for lung cancer, orange is for leukemia (for the full list, search online). Bring on the rainbow.

**The Most Commonly
Diagnosed Cancers in the United States**

(from highest to lowest; source: American Cancer Society, 2015)

1. Breast
2. Lung (including bronchial)
3. Prostate
4. Colon and rectal (combined)
5. Bladder
6. Melanoma
7. Non-Hodgkin's lymphoma
8. Endometrial
9. Leukemia (all types)
10. Kidney (renal cell and renal pelvis)
11. Thyroid
12. Pancreatic

THINK BIG (BUT SMALL)

You have cancer. But your sister is getting married, your daughter is in the school play, you're supposed to attend a work conference in Germany that you've been dreaming about for years. When you get the news, your mind immediately goes to the stuff you think you will miss. Time to redirect your attention.

I tried to balance out my internal to-do list by setting small goals and then bigger ones. My one goal, from the first day of treatment, was to walk my daughter to her classroom the first day of kindergarten. (Ten months later I walked with her to school—very, very slowly, but I made it.) And then I was set on taking a mini-vacation with my family, and then taking a hike to my favorite mountain, and then swimming in the ocean. You might have to adjust the goals as your physical and mental state changes, but keep them in mind as markers and things to look forward to.

CHAPTER 2

SCANS, POKES, AND PRICKS

It should come as no surprise that a cancer diagnosis means you will be touched, examined, scanned, poked, injected, and pricked on a regular basis. You will also become fluent in the language of Cancerland.

SCANS

The nuclear medicine department is one place in Cancerland that you will visit repeatedly. Scans, officially known as medical imaging, are part of the road trip. The main cancer scan lineup includes PET, CT, PET/CT combo, and MRI, each one with its own thrills. Scintigraphy, a type of scan taken of individual organs—such as the kidneys or liver—or bones, could also be in your future. Ultrasounds (sometimes called sonograms) also come into play quite a bit, and throw in mammograms if you're dealing with breast cancer.

Scans are used to determine a diagnosis and staging, then again when deciding on treatment, and during treatment to see if it's working. A radiologist reads the scans, but your oncologist will call you with the results; you won't get them on the day of the scan. (In fact, no one is legally allowed to tell you anything about your scan results except for your physician, so don't bother asking the techs or anyone else.) You show up, get scanned, then go home and wait for a phone call (or sometimes an email if your medical center uses a secure email system). These are outpatient procedures, meaning they don't require a hospital stay. You might have to fast before your scan, which often means no liquids either. Be sure to ask for specifics when you make the appointment. All require that you put on some form of hospital gown, so wear clothes that are easy to get on and off, and don't wear any jewelry or anything with metal in it, including under-wire bras. I always close my eyes during scans, and taking an antianxiety pill an hour before doesn't hurt (your oncologist can write you a prescription for those).

Here's the lowdown on each type of scan you might encounter:

- The PET (POSITRON EMISSION TOMOGRAPHY) SCAN is an imaging scan that looks for disease in the organs and tissues. Because cancerous tissue is more metabolically active, the scan shows any tissue that is different from the normal tissue. Cancerous tumors absorb sugar, so any tumors will light up on the screen. You lie down on a long bench, and an IV of radioactive material (a.k.a. radioisotope injection), or contrast material or dye, is injected in your arm or hand (it could be given orally or rectally instead). The contrast material makes you feel like you're peeing in your pants—as the dye enters your system it warms up the blood, and as it passes through your abdomen area that's the sensation you get. The bench you're lying on slowly moves into the scan machine while you hold your breath in five-second intervals; the whole thing can take thirty to forty minutes (excluding the waiting room backlog).

- The CT (COMPUTED TOMOGRAPHY, SOMETIMES CALLED CAT) SCAN uses X-rays to take images of the body. There are several types, including whole-body CTs. For many abdominal or pelvic CTs you're handed a bottle of an iodine-based or barium sulfate compound to drink one hour before the scan, which acts as a contrast material. And then you wait some more. Sometimes the technicians give you a flavored drink mix like Crystal Light to stir in to make it more palatable. But it's a challenge to keep the liquid down when you're in the middle of treatment. I found drinking it slowly helped, and then chugging the last bit while holding my nose. (If your intestines are getting scanned, you might receive the dye via enema instead.) You're finally led into the scan room, which has two areas: One has the machine and the other holds the booth where the techs run the machine like the Wizard of Oz—you just hear a voice through a speaker (they can see and hear you, in case you need to talk to them). The tech helps you up onto a long bench, and you are slowly rolled into the CT machine, a giant white half-dome that looks like a donut. It takes about twenty to thirty minutes.

- Combination PET/CT (OR PET PLUS CT) SCANS are more common. These use two imaging scans in one procedure: The CT is done first, to take anatomic pictures of the organs, and then the PET scan looks at chemical changes in tissue. Before the scan you have to drink a contrast material and wait thirty minutes. Then you're led into another room where a tech preps you for an IV of contrast dye, usually made of glucose. After that, it's off to the actual scan room. You lie down on a bench, the tech connects the IV—usually in your hand or arm—and you're slowly rolled into the machine. The contrast dye starts flowing and, again, it feels like you're peeing your pants. You have to hold your breath for a few seconds, and then you're done. The whole thing takes under five minutes. Drink a lot of water afterward to flush your kidneys; the techs usually tell you to avoid alcohol and caffeine for six to eight hours. I always bring crackers or nuts to eat afterward because I always feel a little sick to my stomach after all that stuff has been flowing through me.

- The MRI (MAGNETIC RESONANCE IMAGING) uses a magnet and radio waves—rather than radiation or X-rays—to look at your insides. The magnet stimulates activity in the cells and can capture these signals on a computer screen and produce a three-dimensional image of the body; it's particularly useful for looking at soft tissue. The machine is tunnel-shaped, and you slide into it on a sliding bed; the noise it emits sounds like someone is banging a hammer on the side of the wall next to your head. It doesn't hurt or involve any liquids. It's a more expensive scan for the hospital than a PET, CT, or X-ray.

- SCINTIGRAPHY is a two-dimensional test that uses a camera and computer to produce images called scintigrams. The patient is given a radioisotope injection, and the scanner traces the gamma rays present in the radioisotopes. Any areas where cells are repairing themselves—sometimes called "hot spots"—take up the most amount of tracer and indicate where there is injury or disease. Each type of scintigraphy has its own name (skeletal scintigraphy is the official term for a bone scan, for example, and renal scintigraphy is a kidney scan). I've had four bone scans, and it's an easy, painless process. You get the IV injection, and depending on the body part being scanned, you are either scanned immediately or you may have to wait between two and four hours for the radioisotopes to move into your bloodstream. When it's time for the actual scan, you lie down on the table and hold still while the scanner goes up and down your body. A full-body scan takes about twenty minutes. Drink lots of water afterward to help flush the injection material out of your body; the only way to get it out is through urinating. (It takes two days for it to be eliminated completely.)

Be sure to request a copy of the scan for your records as soon as you can, while you're signing in or immediately after the scan. The check-in desks usually have imagery request forms and can have the CD with the scans ready for you that day (ask the hospital for the specific form). I can't say it enough: Get your own copies of everything. Each doctor and hospital will ask for the scans, and waiting for one doctor to send something to another (a town or state or country away) on your behalf can be like waiting for Godot.

I've had so many scans that I sometimes had to ask the tech which scan I was there for. You'll be scanned most often just after your initial diagnosis, when they are trying to determine where exactly the cancer has spread and how far it has progressed. And you never know what scans you might need. About six months after my diagnosis I had to get a brain MRI, "just to cross it off the list" and make sure there was no brain swelling causing my nausea. I spent thirty-five minutes in the MRI machine with a "lid" on my head (basically a giant hockey mask strapped across my face). With the aid of calming drugs, I daydreamed about a hilltop in Italy and got through it. At some point, much later, I laughed. Brain cancer?! Wasn't one mortal dilemma enough?

There are also what I call "side" scans and tests that might be required. For example, before you receive Adriamycin, a chemotherapy drug, you might need a scan to check your heart. The drug can damage heart muscle, so the oncologist needs to be sure your heart is healthy enough to withstand it.

Personalized Medicine and Genetic Testing

PERSONALIZED MEDICINE

The newest scientific approach in oncology treatment is called personalized, or precision, medicine. It is an approach that allows doctors to create personal therapies based on the genomes and molecular structure of the specific cancer. This is a very important breakthrough for cancer patients, because traditionally doctors would try the same therapies on all patients and then switch to other drugs if the tumor continued to grow (what the FDA calls the "one-dose-fits-all" approach).

But with personalized medicine, doctors can start with a specific treatment that has a very specific rationale for an individual patient based on that patient's cancer. These targeted therapies or treatments have been effective against numerous types of cancer, including colorectal, kidney, breast, lung, and melanoma. The federal government supported this approach by announcing funding and launching the Precision Medicine Initiative in 2015, with research funded through the National Cancer Institute and several other government agencies.

GENETIC TESTING

We are all born with a set of genes—our eye color, hair color, and certain types of disease can be linked to genetics. Cancer is caused by genes that have been damaged—called "oncogenes"— because of a defective gene (genetic mutation), such as BRCA1 or BRCA2, from environmental effects such as smoking, or from just having worn out with age. When the cells that should be at rest begin to divide and develop into a tumor, cancer occurs.

The biggest genetic breakthrough in ovarian and breast cancer came in 1994 when the genetic coding for BCRA1 and BRCA2 were discovered, making it possible to identify families and individual patients in these families who are at very high risk for breast and ovarian cancers. After many years of research, specific chemotherapies were developed that are especially effective in breast and ovarian cancer patients who tested positive for mutant forms of these genes. In 1998 the chemotherapy drug Herceptin (trastuzumab) was approved for use in HER2-positive breast cancer patients. HER2 is a gene that goes out of control in about 25 percent of breast cancers; the gene makes too many copies of itself, which leads to cancer. (This discovery was one of the earliest steps in targeted medicine.) BRCA1, BRCA2, and HER2 are examples of biomarkers that are used to detect, diagnose, and treat some cancers.

Genetic testing (or genomic analysis, in medical-speak) is now part of every cancer diagnosis. Many medical centers have genetic counselors on staff that will meet with you to discuss the test results and options.

If you are a high-risk individual (because of ethnic background or family history, among other factors) but haven't been diagnosed with cancer, schedule an appointment with a genetic counselor—the National Society of Genetic Counselors (NSGC) provides a list (see Resources for more information). Some doctors are advocating testing for high-risk patients before the average age of testing, which is often quite late (forty and older). Some geneticists are advocating testing at age thirty. (BRCA1 and BRCA2 can be inherited from both the maternal and paternal sides of the family.)

Deciding whether and when to get tested can be stressful, particularly if you have siblings and other family members who might be affected by the results. (In my case, I was worried about both my mother and my sister, as well as my daughter and my son, who can't be tested until they're twenty-one.) But don't skip genetic testing because of fear of losing your job or any other type of discrimination. The federal Genetic Information Nondiscrimination Act (GINA) of 2008 protects you from job discrimination and health care coverage discrimination due to any genetic testing results. Likewise, cost shouldn't stop you from getting tested—the cost of genetic testing has gone down significantly (in some cases, about 75 percent) in part because of a 2013 US Supreme Court decision (*Association for Molecular Pathology v. Myriad Genetics*) that banned the patenting of certain genes.

Even though genetic testing has come down in cost, it can still be expensive, and insurance doesn't always pay for it. Still, genetic testing is now part of the American medical landscape—a 2012 study by the UnitedHealth Group found that $5 billion was spent on genetic testing in 2010.

POKES & PRICKS

Having cancer means blood tests—blood draws or blood work in medical-speak—and dozens and dozens (dare I say hundreds?) of pricks. The first thing to say about blood work: It's never convenient. It's either an early-morning appointment or the laboratory line is so long you end up waiting for an hour.

If possible, schedule any blood work or scans for early in the morning. That way you won't have to starve yourself all day (since they often require fasting), and usually the waiting room isn't as crowded. It's just like airports: The later you go, the more backlog you'll encounter. I used to schedule 7:00 AM blood draws and 8:00 AM scans, and then reward myself afterwards with a big stack of pancakes at the local diner. (See Chemo 101 in chapter 4 for more on scheduling.)

Watching vials of blood being drawn from your arm starts out as a perhaps-painful curiosity and then becomes as routine as brushing your teeth. First of all, learn the names of the people who are drawing your blood: They are called phlebotomists. You will get to know the best techs, the ones who do it effortlessly and painlessly, and the best veins. (I didn't know this, but not all veins are created equal.)

Traditionally blood is drawn from the inside of your arm near your elbow (called the antecubital area). If you are sensitive on the inside of your arms, try the back of your hands (this is my preferred method now that I am port-free; see Vein or Port? in chapter 4 for more on ports). If no vein is available in your arms, the tech will draw from the veins in the top of your feet (this is rare, though). They wrap a plastic band (tourniquet) around your arm while you make a fist so blood flows into the vein; there is an alcohol swab, a prick, tourniquet comes off, and you unclench your fist. If you're prone to fainting or light-headedness around blood or needles, tell the technician beforehand.

The plastic vials of blood are capped, a piece of gauze and sticky tape is stuck on your arm, and you're done. (If you've got kids who've turned their dolls into proxies for you, ask for extra neon-colored medical tape so they can play doctor at home.) Wear long sleeves to cover up the gauze and the rainbow-colored bruises that will form, and wear a loose-fitting top with sleeves you can easily pull up to reveal your veins. I'll never forget my first real day as a patient, before I knew the ropes. I wore a black long-sleeved shirt with a black vest and black pants and boots. Was I trying to out-fashion my cancer? Not the best choice for undergoing tests and getting dressed and undressed ten times as I made my way around the medical center.

The blood draws will take longer if you have a PICC line or a port (see the next section for more on both)—not every tech is qualified to draw blood with these methods.

At some point, patient life is just one poke after another. One afternoon my mom and I went to a matinee to kill time between medical "events"; all through the movie our cell phones kept buzzing. We ignored them till we couldn't anymore. Of the dozens of texts awaiting us, I read my husband's first: "I know you're in the movies. Please leave now because you have to get blood drawn before the lab closes in 15 minutes." I sighed, put down the M&Ms, and we headed for the hospital.

CANCERSPEAK, PART 2: A GUIDE TO MEDICAL TERMS YOU WILL HEAR OVER AND OVER (AND OVER AGAIN)

Use this guide to learn the terminology and decipher all the letters—the medical community loves an acronym!

- ADJUVANT THERAPY: Any therapy (as in, a drug) that is given in conjunction with another therapy to help its efficacy. In relation to chemotherapy, "adjuvant chemo" refers to chemo given after cancer surgery.

- ADVANCE MEDICAL DIRECTIVE (AMD): A legal form that states your medical wishes and names the person you would like to make medical decisions for you. The form varies by state but usually includes a section for power of attorney and another section for things like donation of organs. A completed AMD is often a mandatory part of your hospital patient file before any procedure or surgery. Also known as an advance directive or living will, it can be revoked at any time. (A health care proxy or HCP is a type of AMD; for more information see The Big Talks: Wills and Advance Medical Directives in chapter 9.)

- ANALGESIC: A medication, topical or oral, that relieves pain.

- ANTIEMETIC: A type of drug used to control nausea and vomiting, often prescribed with chemotherapy.

- BENIGN: A term used to describe cells that are abnormal but cannot spread to other parts of the body or invade nearby tissue. Often they can simply be removed.

- BIOPSY: A sample of tissue taken from the body for further study; most often used to detect cancer. There are many, many types of biopsies, and some of them involve removing tissue with a needle. Common cancer biopsies include the fine-needle biopsy, core biopsy (which uses a larger needle than a fine-needle biopsy), liver biopsy, and skin biopsy. The tissue is then reviewed under a microscope by a pathologist. The results of the biopsy can take minutes (such as during surgery) or a few days. Some biopsies are done in doctors' offices, while others are done under CT scan or by ultrasound in hospitals or medical centers.

- BRCA1: A gene on chromosome 17 that normally helps cells protect their DNA from damage. People who inherit mutations to this gene have a higher risk of breast, ovarian, prostate, and other cancers. BRCA testing is now performed on patients diagnosed with breast cancer and can also be done on high-risk people starting at around age twenty-one. The test comes back as BRCA positive or negative: Positive means you have the genetic mutation and negative means you don't. Genetic counseling is prescribed for people who are BRCA1- or BRCA2-positive. (See the sidebar earlier in this chapter for more on genetic testing.)

- BRCA2: A gene on chromosome 13 that normally helps cells protect their DNA from damage. People who inherit mutations to this gene have a higher risk of breast, ovarian, prostate, and other cancers. (See the sidebar earlier in this chapter for more on genetic testing.)

- CANCER: A term, per the American Cancer Society, used to describe "more than 100 different diseases in which cells grow out of control."

- CANDIDATE: This means you. No, you're not running for political office. In the medical world, "candidate" means you the patient, as in, "a candidate for surgery." As in, you are eligible or you qualify for x, y, or z.

- CBC: Complete blood count, a term used by the doctor when he or she orders blood work.

- CHARGE NURSE: The nurse in charge of the department at the hospital during his or her shift.

- CHEMOTHERAPY: Often called "chemo" among patients and written as "CT" in your medical chart, the term refers to drug treatment that destroys cancer cells. (For more on chemotherapy, see chapter 4.)

- CINV: Chemotherapy-induced nausea and vomiting. The official medical phrase for the nausea and vomiting experienced after a cycle of chemo.

- CLEAR MARGINS: Refers to surgical margins, also known as a negative margin. It means the doctors found no linked cancer cells at the edge of the tissue removed during surgery, which indicates that the surgical resection successfully removed all the contiguous cancer. Unlike most cancer terminology, in this case "negative" is a good thing. The other types of margins are positive margins (meaning cancer cells were found at the edge of the resected tissue sample; this is not good news) and close margins (somewhere between positive and negative).

- COCKTAIL: Shorthand for "chemo cocktail," or a combination of chemotherapy drugs.

- COMPASSIONATE USE (ALSO "EXPANDED ACCESS"): Refers to experimental (or investigational) drugs made available to patients outside of a clinical trial (who are not in a trial or need to get into a closed trial), or a clinical trial drug that is in a later stage that may be given to a patient who doesn't qualify for the trial. To be considered for compassionate use, your doctor contacts the drug manufacturer and submits an application to the FDA, then the FDA makes a decision. (Unless your situation is dire or considered an emergency, there is no set timeline on how long you will wait to get an answer.) The concept of expanded access began under the FDA in 1987. Complete eligibility guidelines, requirements, and information are on the FDA's website (www.fda.gov—search for "expanded access" or "compassionate use").

- CYTOTOXIN: A substance that prevents cells from reproducing and/or that destroys cells.

- EHR: Electronic health record. The electronic version of a patient's medical record.

- EKG: Electrocardiogram, a test used to determine the electrical function of your heart (the body has a natural electrical system that keeps the heart muscle pumping). The test is performed while you lie on a table, and electrodes are attached to areas of your body using an electrode paste. You lie still, sometimes holding your breath, while the heart activity is transmitted. It takes no more than ten minutes and is a completely safe, painless test. (EKG equipment is portable so it can be moved around, rather than you having to go to a particular room or area of the medical center.)

- FINE NEEDLE ASPIRATION (FNA): A type of biopsy where a thin needle is inserted into the tissue. You're awake during the procedure and it hurts like hell, but it's very standard and safe.

- FIRST-LINE THERAPY: Also known as first-line treatment, it's the first treatment given to the patient to eliminate disease. Usually the first-line therapy is part of a sequence of therapies. For example, first-line therapy for breast cancer may be chemotherapy followed by surgery and then radiation therapy.

- FISH (FLUORESCENCE IN SITU HYBRIDIZATION): A test used to "map" certain genes in cancer cells. It can also be used to determine how responsive a patient will be to chemotherapy. It's commonly used in breast cancer, bladder cancer, and certain types of leukemia diagnoses. It examines tissue to see abnormalities that are too small to see under a microscope. The test may or may not be covered by your health insurance.

- GRAY (GY): A unit used to measure the amount of radiation absorbed by human tissue.

- HEALTH INSURANCE PORTABILITY AND ACCOUNTABILITY ACT (HIPPA): A federal law passed in 1996. Covers portability (meaning continuity of care, which is now part of the Affordable Care Act) and privacy. The privacy aspect is constantly referenced in the medical world and it basically says no medical personnel can discuss your medical information with anyone except for you, a person or persons you designate, and other medical staff members assigned to your care. HIPPA is taken extremely seriously.

- HERCEPTIN: A type of chemotherapy drug used on patients with cancers that have tested positive for the HER2 gene. Also known as trastuzumab, Herceptin is a relatively new drug (it was developed in the 1990s) and has been successful in treating both HER2-positive breast cancer patients and, more recently, stomach cancer patients.

- HICKMAN LINE: Similar to the PICC line, it's a central catheter that is threaded into the jugular vein and goes directly to the heart. Used for chemotherapy treatment.

- HODGKIN'S LYMPHOMA (HL): Cancer of the lymph glands, named after Thomas Hodgkin, a British anatomist who first noticed swelling in the glands of male cadavers. This type of cancer spreads locally, from one lymph node to another. Non-Hodgkin's lymphoma (NHL) is a similar cancer that originates in a different type of white blood cell called a lymphocyte. NHL is among the top ten most common cancers in the United States, according to the National Cancer Institute.

- HORMONE REPLACEMENT THERAPY (HRT OR HT; ALSO CALLED MENOPAUSAL HORMONE THERAPY OR MHT): Refers to a type of treatment where menopausal women are given hormones (estrogen and/or progesterone) to replace those that are no longer produced by the ovaries. This treatment is sometimes prescribed for female cancer patients that have had their ovaries removed or if their ovaries are damaged, which requires artificial hormones. Usually dispensed in tablet form. (For more on HRT, see Recurrence in chapter 12.)

- INFLAMMATORY BREAST CANCER (IBC): A rare, aggressive form of breast cancer with few symptoms that tends to affect younger women. The cancer cells attack the skin and lymph vessels of the breast. Once the lymph vessels become blocked, some symptoms—such as an orange peel–like texture, redness and swelling on the breast, or dimpled or flattened nipples—start to appear. IBC accounts for about 1 to 5 percent of all breast cancers in the United States every year, according to the National Cancer Institute.

- INFUSION: A method of giving medication through a vein with a pump rather than with a syringe.

- LEUKEMIA: A broad term to describe cancer of the blood system, which begins in the bone marrow. There are nine major types of leukemia.

- LOCALLY ADVANCED CANCER: Refers to a cancer that has spread from the original tumor site to the surrounding tissue or lymph nodes.

- LUMPECTOMY (LX): The removal of a breast tumor (lump) and a small amount of surrounding tissue. Also called partial mastectomy, it is not as invasive as mastectomy, and the shape of the breast and nipple are usually retained. Often performed as an outpatient procedure with local or general anesthesia. You will be sore and possibly numb after the procedure.

- LYMPHOSCINTIGRAPHY: An exam done in the hospital's nuclear medicine department before the removal of the sentinel lymph node(s). (A sentinel lymph node is "the first lymph node to which cancer cells are most likely to spread from a primary tumor," according to the National Cancer Institute. There can be more than one sentinel lymph node.) A tiny amount of radioactive material (called a tracer) is injected into your arm through an IV and, as the material moves through the lymphatic channels, the scan shows which lymph nodes are at risk for containing cancer cells. The procedure takes about one hour. You lie down on a table, and a technician moves a camera around your body taking images; it doesn't hurt except for some soreness at the injection point. (For more on scintigraphy, see Scans at the beginning of this chapter.)

- MALIGNANT: A word used to describe a cancerous tumor that is made up of cells that are dividing out of control and spreading. Malignant tumors may or may not be operable.

- MAMMOGRAM: An X-ray of the breast. A bilateral mammogram is the term when both breasts are X-rayed; unilateral is the term for when only one breast is.

- MASS: A word used to describe abnormal tissue; used interchangeably with the words "tumor," "neoplasm," and "lesion."

- MASTECTOMY (MX): The surgical removal of the breast and surrounding tissue. Considered a major surgery with an overnight hospital stay required and performed under general anesthesia. Double mastectomy refers to the removal of both breasts. Numbness in the chest area is a common side effect and is often permanent. The first mastectomy was performed in 1882 by Dr. William Halsted, an American surgeon who pioneered the procedure now called the radical mastectomy, which removed the breast, lymphatic tissue, and the pectoralis muscle.

- METASTASIS: Refers to a secondary cancer, which occurs when a malignant tumor moves away from the primary cancer site and spreads to other areas of the body. The word means "beyond stillness" in Latin. Metastases is the plural form, abbreviated as "mets."

- MRN (MEDICAL RECORD NUMBER): An identifying patient number, usually used in larger medical centers.

- NED (NO EVIDENCE OF DISEASE): This is determined by tests and examinations and indicates that the patient who has been treated for cancer has no evidence of disease. The equivalent of remission, it can be temporary or permanent. (You want to hear this term.)

- NEUROPATHY: Describes damage to the nerves. It can be named after a specific disease or after specific types of nerves. Cancer patients often experience peripheral

neuropathy, which manifests as pain that is tingling and/
or burning, or weakness in the hands and feet due to
damaged peripheral nerves. It's a common side effect of
chemotherapy and radiation. It can also be caused by the
tumor itself—for example, tumors can put pressure on
nerves and cause pain. Talk to your doctor immediately
if you have any tingling pain. (See Chemo Side Effects in
chapter 4 for more on neuropathy.)

- NEOADJUVANT CHEMOTHERAPY: Chemotherapy given
  before surgery in order to shrink the tumor.

- NODE-NEGATIVE: Cancer that has not spread to the
  lymph nodes.

- NPO: Instructions for the patient to take nothing by
  mouth (usually before surgery or before certain blood
  tests). Stands for the Latin *non per os* or *nil per os* meaning
  "nothing by mouth."

- NUCLEAR MEDICINE: A branch of radiology that uses
  radioactive tracers and a special camera to diagnose disease
  in human tissue. The most common type is the PET scan.

- ONCOTYPE DX (ALSO CALLED ONCO, OR 21-GENE
  SIGNATURE): A type of test performed on certain breast
  cancer patients to help determine the course of treatment.
  The test uses tissue taken from a biopsy or surgery and
  looks at twenty-one different genes within the cancer cell.

- OOP: Out of pocket, usually referring to costs incurred by
  patients with insurance that are not covered by the health
  insurance company.

- OOPHORECTOMY: The removal of one or both of the ovaries. If the fallopian tubes are removed as well, it's called a salpingo-oophorectomy.

- OTC: Over-the-counter, referring to medications you can buy without a prescription.

- OUTCOME: In the medical world, "survival outcome" refers to whether you live or die. Positive outcome means the patient lives; negative outcome means the patient died. It is also used to describe whether the patient had a recurrence of cancer or not. The term isn't inherently negative; there is also "disease-free outcome."

- PALLIATIVE THERAPY: Care that is intended to work with other therapies to ease the side effects of cancer treatment. (For more on palliative care, see Chemo 101 in chapter 4.)

- PATHOLOGY: The description of a patient's tissue sample, which can include the size, grade, and type of tumor and tumor marker.

- PATH REPORT: Short for pathology report, a medical document prepared by a pathologist after a biopsy or surgery. The pathologist gives the report to your oncologist, who then gives you the information. A pathologist is a doctor who specializes in examining blood, tissue, or bodily fluids.

- PHLEBOTOMIST: A technician who performs blood draws.

- PICC (PERIPHERALLY INSERTED CENTRAL CATHETER) LINE: A long, thin tube that is threaded directly through a vein in the arm so the tip rests near the heart. It's basically an IV line that stays open to deliver infusions and withdraw blood samples. The line sticks out of your arm and is sealed and wrapped in gauze; it must be cleaned by a nurse in a doctor's office once a week, which takes about five minutes. A nurse must insert the PICC line, which takes about twenty minutes. Having it removed involves one quick pull by another nurse. PICC lines are not waterproof, and you have to be careful that nothing—kid, dog—yanks on it or pulls it out. The general medical consensus is that the PICC line is safer than the Hickman line because it has less risk of infection.

- PORT: Also called a portacath. A catheter about the size of a quarter is surgically inserted under the collarbone and then used for infusions. A very standard outpatient procedure. An interventional radiologist performs it while you're awake but numbed. The recovery takes one week. (When I received my chest port I felt like I had been kicked in the chest by a horse.) The port is accessed with a Huber needle, which basically punctures the port—it feels like a sharp, long bee sting. You can feel the port under your skin, but it isn't a tube dangling from your arm like the PICC line. I grew to love my port; it never has to be cleaned, and I found it much easier than the PICC line (although slightly more painful to access). And they're waterproof, so you can swim and shower without having to worry about infection. And it saves your veins if you have to receive months of IV drugs—over time veins may start to collapse (see

Vein or Port? in chapter 4 for more about veins). Blood can also be drawn from the port.

- PSA (PROSTATE-SPECIFIC ANTIGEN): A substance produced by the prostate gland; a blood test revealing higher-than-usual levels of PSA in men can indicate the presence of prostate cancer. Amounts are measured in ng/mL, or nanograms per milliliter. Men should discuss the pros and cons of prostate cancer screening with their doctors.

- RBC (RED BLOOD CELL COUNT): Red blood cell count, measured through a blood sample.

- REMISSION: According to the National Cancer Institute, *remission* means "a decrease in or disappearance of signs and symptoms of cancer. In partial remission, some, but not all, signs and symptoms of cancer have disappeared. In complete remission, all signs and symptoms of cancer have disappeared, although cancer still may be in the body."

- SARCOMA: A malignant tumor that grows on connective tissue such as fat, cartilage, bone, or muscle.

- STAGE: How far the cancer has progressed in the body, ranging from Stage 0 through Stage IV—0 being the best and IV the worst. Each type of cancer is staged according to specific factors: Generally, the stage is determined by the size of the tumor, the number of lymph nodes involved, and whether there are signs that the cancer has spread to other parts of the body. In breast cancer, ductal carcimona in situ (DCIS), now known as Stage 0, refers to abnormal cells found in the lining of milk-producing ducts. This is far more prevalent in young women and accounts for about 60,000 cases of breast cancer in the United States every year.

- STANDING ORDER: An order requested by your physician that refers to a recurring test, such as a weekly blood draw.

- STAT: An abbreviation in medical centers meaning "immediately"; from the Latin word *statim*, meaning "at once." Usually written in all capital letters.

- SUBCUTANEOUS (SC, SQ): Refers to administering medications just below the surface of the skin (rather than by IV or catheter).

- TAMOXIFEN: A type of medication called an antiestrogen, which comes in tablet form and is prescribed for a certain type of breast cancer patient as hormone therapy. It works by blocking estrogen receptors in breast tissue and is effective in ER-positive breast cancer patients. (Also known as Nolvadex.)

- THERAPY: This isn't the "talk-out-your-problems" kind of therapy. In oncology, *therapy* refers to treatment (as in, chemotherapy and radiation therapy).

- TRIPLE-NEGATIVE: Refers to a specific type of breast cancer where the three main receptors that are thought to "fuel" most tumors—estrogen, progesterone, and the HER2 gene—are not present in the tumor. In this case, "negative" isn't good; it's actually the opposite. Fifteen percent of all breast cancer in the United States is triple-negative, according to the National Breast Cancer Foundation.

- TUMOR: A growth of abnormal tissue that is uncontrolled and may be solid or filled with fluid; also known as a neoplasm. In general, a tumor is caused by a group of cells that are dividing excessively.

- VITALS: Abbreviation for vital signs, which are blood pressure, oxygenation, respiration, heart rate, and temperature. Your vitals—often along with your height and weight— are taken by a nurse at every medical appointment.

- WBC (WHITE BLOOD CELL COUNT): White blood cell count, measured through a blood sample.

CHAPTER 3

ATTITUDE

The word *attitude* gets thrown around a lot with cancer patients, as if only those of us with a positive attitude will prevail. I find it offensive. No one can possibly "stay positive" through every second of the road trip. The trick is to stay mostly positive while you feel and sort through the rest of the stuff. If emotions are ruling your world right now, this is the chapter for you.

FEAR

For most people, the companion word to *cancer* is *fear*. It's inescapable and only natural. The word *cancer* has been used in American culture not only as a medical diagnosis but also as an awful, negative term for anything worthy of disdain, and even for things that are considered evil. The "C-word" has been haunting patients since the 1800s when doctors still whispered it and patients were afraid to tell their family and friends. Some cultures still to this day do not discuss the C-word in mixed company. (Susan Sontag wrote about this so wonderfully in her classic, illuminating work, *Illness as Metaphor*.)

Fearing for your life, fearing for the people around you—there are endless forms of fear that emerge when you're handed the news. It's a strange thing to fear this cell, this disease—something you can't see with the naked eye but that has invaded your body while you were driving, eating breakfast, or typing up a quarterly report for your boss. For me, the fear was rooted in the unknown: what was to come in treatment, and even worse, what the ultimate outcome would be. As I started treatment I also became fearful of believing too strongly in any one medication or procedure; I felt like the goalposts kept changing. So I was afraid to feel hopeful. At times it was pure terror, wondering what could happen. And fear can be paralyzing. At some point—for me, it was about five months in—you have to release it. It's too exhausting to be afraid all of the time, physically and emotionally.

I broke my fears down into two lists, which might save you some time and heartache: What is actually scary and what is just your mind pulling you around.

Things to Fear

When you have cancer, these are the things I think are reasonable to be afraid of:

- Getting sick from people coughing, germy kids, and dirty grocery store shopping cart handles.

- The remote controls and light switches in hotel rooms. Always wipe them down with alcohol wipes.

- Dying.

- Hospital food. (Always pack your own or get family or friends to bring food in.)

- Chatty patients and/or relatives in waiting and treatment rooms.

- People who look away when they talk to you.

- Insensitive comments.

- Crying in front of your kids.

- A lack of pain relief. If you're in pain, speak up. You are your best advocate.

- Your plastic surgeon asking you in the pre-op room to remind them what size breasts you wanted.

- Taking the first answer you get. (It will always be no.)

- People avoiding you. Even people you thought were close friends.

- Asking, "Why me?" It's a black hole of a question—it's unanswerable and just makes you miserable.

- Believing that everything you thought was true and good may be wrong.

- Watching your old life end.

Things Not to Fear

Things that are overblown, exaggerated, or not as scary as they seem:

- Being bald.

- Being old.

- Being loud.

- Dancing in the streets. Literally.

- Asking questions.

- Eating dessert first. (And ordering a double scoop.)

- Saying the word *breast* (or *colon*, or *prostate*, or *testicle*) out loud. Over and over again.

- Clinical drug trials. I swore up and down that I would never be a guinea pig, a rat, an experiment, and exactly two months later I was begging, begging to get into a trial. (See Clinical Trials in chapter 4 for more.)

- Seeing a shrink (psychiatrist, psychologist, therapist, or counselor). Therapy might be what you need right now, and you can find a mental health professional (or religious or spiritual advisor) that you vibe with. It's particularly helpful if you can find one that specializes in oncology patients. They are the ones you can call when you feel everyone around you is "cancered out," when you need to talk about the fact that you've been dealt a shitty hand.

- Complaining, when appropriate. Send back a bad meal; life is too short!

- Lows. The lowest lows have to end sometime, and a high is just around the corner. The darkness will end, but you have to stick it out.

- Doing something unexpected, whether it's offering an opinion, asking someone a difficult question, or taking that extra drive to look out at the mountains.

- Calling your surgeon the day before surgery to be sure he or she knows you want saline, not silicone, breast implants.

- Taking one last good look at your _____ (insert body part) before surgery.

- Planning a future.

- Writing a letter to your kids and/or your spouse, partner, or other family members, even if they never read it.

- Talking about dying.

- Explaining to your closest friends just how afraid you are.

- Taking a luxurious trip, even if it's one night. Be sure it includes room service.

- Other people's emotional baggage.

- Asking your surgeon(s) if they got a good night's sleep.

- Playing the "cancer card."

- Speaking up when you've been waiting to get a mammogram or an ultrasound for more than thirty minutes and you're in pain and goddamn it can you just be moved to the front of the line, in front of the cranky lady who won't stop talking and who's just having a routine mammogram?

- Smiling. It sounds horrific—like the worst Hallmark card ever—but during a low point when you can't seem to drag your sorry ass out of bed or move from the pain, try to crack a smile. At the very least it might lead to a little laughter.

- Getting an eyebrow wax or a manicure and pedicure. If you're up for it, indulge. Some oncologists advise you to avoid mani/pedis because of infection risk (I wasn't allowed to get them for about a year), but I did keep what remained of my eyebrows in tip-top shape. When you're bald those brows stand out, and damned if I was going to be a cancer patient with a unibrow. (For more on beauty tips and resources, see Slap On a Little Lipstick in chapter 8.)

- Buying a pretty shirt, or a pair of heels, or some ridiculously expensive running shoes. (I bought myself some kick-ass cowboy boots while killing time between oncology appointments in Houston. I treasure them.) While your body may be bloated from chemo and assorted drugs, your feet hopefully won't change (although anything is possible with the Big C). It's amazing what one small, beautiful thing can do to lift your spirits.

The Big D

Acknowledging the possibility of death doesn't make you negative; it makes you human. And in a culture where death is hardly discussed anyway, it makes sense that it would be a hard topic to face, either personally or communally.

Hospice refers to a team that provides medical care, pain

management, and social and emotional support for patients with terminal illnesses. If hospice looks like it might be a part of this road trip, ask your caregiver to research it just like any other resource and talk to your medical team (The National Hospice and Palliative Care Organization is the best place to start; see Resources).

Whether or not your prognosis leads to hospice, it's important to think about end-of-life issues such as pain management, organ donation, and burial/funeral arrangements and get your wishes in writing. Again, if your family and/or caregivers are uncomfortable discussing these topics, find someone you can trust who can and will help you write it down.

HOPE

Flip fear over and you'll find hope. The word *hope* gets thrown around medical centers and plastered across T-shirts, mugs, and greeting cards. Maybe because it's an approachable word—it has less religious connotation than the word *believe*, for example. For whatever reason, I embraced it. It was something to keep my spirits up, and it wasn't as frustrating as words like *fight*. (Of course you're fighting; that's supposed to be inspiration?) My dear artist friend made a beautiful vase with HOPE written across it; it sat next to my bed, and I looked at it a hundred times each day. I feel like hope is an emotion that can keep you floating when you are in dark seas, and I used it as a life raft even when scans came back with bad news or my blood counts remained uncooperatively low. The words THERE IS ALWAYS HOPE stand in large lettering across the front of the City of Hope Medical

Center, and I took that to heart every single time I walked through the doors.

OTHER PEOPLE'S HOPES AND FEARS

Remember that your family is your family whether you are sick or not. The same disagreements, resentments, habits, and behavior that existed before you were diagnosed are still there. Did your brother always take charge when you were younger? He will probably try to take charge of your illness. Your sister never hugged you growing up? She won't start now. They have their own fears and hopes and feelings about your illness. And your family might not want to talk about it. Or, they might want to talk about it all the time. Accepting them either way is the tricky part. It's easy to say it, easy to suggest it, but when you're deep in treatment all of the emotional stuff can be overwhelming.

It's up to you to set boundaries you're comfortable with. If your brother drives you to chemo and his driving makes you anxious, or your mother plans to spend every night with you while you "get through this" when you'd rather she stay with your aunt, get ready to talk about it. Hashing things out can be difficult to do, particularly if you and everyone around you are aware that you might not make it. Why fight when time is precious? But aside from having a terminal, six-months-to-live diagnosis that would allow you to let it all unfold however you damn well please, there will be a time (probably seven weeks after your diagnosis) when you, your family, and your caregivers need to have a sit-down and figure out a few ground rules. I noticed my support system's patience waned and attitudes changed slightly at the seven-week mark; the shock and awe had worn off a bit, and everyone realized this would be a longer haul than originally anticipated. And fatigue had probably set in. It turns out there is a term for this: the "shelf life of compassion."

It's ideal if you can all sit down in a room together (or Skype, video conference, or however you can all gather) and talk about the next month or two and how everyone can help get you through it. Use the time to set specific parameters for what makes you comfortable. If your mother won't stop chatting to the oncology nurse and that makes you insane, ask a friend or another relative to come with you to chemo. You don't have to be rude about it; there are ways to get your needs met without alienating your loved ones. And this conversation is absolutely crucial if there are children in the mix: setting a routine for them must be a priority (for more on this, see Parenting with Cancer in chapter 9).

In the midst of all these people (your partner, family, friends, medical team), you might still feel lonely. Because ultimately this is your road trip, your body, and your life. I was surprised by the sense of isolation I often felt. Although there may be people who help make everyday life easier, you're the one whose veins are poked, whose body is filling up with chemo drugs, and who is being radiated until you can hardly move.

Bucket Lists

Something that cheered me up during the rough moments was dreaming about what I would do—both alone and with my family—when it was "over." I made wild lists, not necessarily based on reality, but it was fun to dream and even more fun to look through them when I was feeling better. I typed, I wrote in notebooks, I browsed real estate on my iPad, I collected magazine clippings. Dreaming of a Hawaiian vacation, a cruise to Alaska, a golf trip, or a Vegas getaway might get you through a tough week or even a difficult month. Plan that trip to the very last detail; it will set your mind in another, lovely direction. Very few of the things on my outlandish wish list—grand redecorating plans, adventure trips to Peru—ended up happening (yet!), but it was the planning process that pulled me through. I could hear the sound of the ocean, I could feel the warm sand on my feet, and that was enough to get me thinking ahead instead of staring at the bottles and bottles of pills that lined the top of our dresser.

It also helped to make a list with the kids. My daughter Penelope was old enough to be able to think of the immediate future, so we would make small lists of attainable trips or activities (like taking the ferry to San Francisco or getting towering ice cream sundaes at Ghirardelli Chocolate Factory) that made the weeks more bearable. Take the kids to an amusement park; let the sticky cotton candy cling to your fingers and your lips; listen to the screams of the people on the roller coaster. Buy them popcorn and a roll of tickets and go wild. The little things matter now more than ever.

NAVIGATING THE RIVER OF DENIAL AND OTHER EMOTIONAL ROLLERCOASTERS

The explosion of emotions that I felt after my diagnosis had no rhyme or reason. I felt extremely disoriented during those first weeks. You might feel caught off guard, particularly if you were living a healthy lifestyle or were rarely sick and thought that would keep the Big C at bay.

Elisabeth Kübler-Ross, who so brilliantly wrote about death, dying, and grieving, is credited with establishing the five stages of death that she then applied to grief in *On Grief and Grieving: Finding the Meaning of Grief Through the Five Stages of Loss.* The stages arrive in no particular order, and you might experience one, two, or all five of them. Being aware of them might help you through the process. (Kübler-Ross also writes about anticipatory grief, which can occur months or even years before a death. Caretakers can feel this acutely while watching a loved one struggle, or patients who have been given a serious diagnosis might experience it. It's something to bring up with a therapist or mental health professional.)

The five stages of grief Kübler-Ross describes are, in no particular order:

- Denial

- Anger

- Bargaining

- Depression

- Acceptance

In retrospect, I realize I grieved my own illness for the first few months after I was diagnosed, and then I grieved again during different stages of treatment. Denial arrived first, with many days beginning with my mind thinking it was all a dream, that it wasn't really happening. Bargaining was a major player: the cliché "If you let me live I will do x, y, and z." (Yes, I thought that many times.)

Guilt also came in and out fairly steadily throughout the first year. I felt guilty for causing everyone so much trouble, worry, and money; I felt "mom guilt" for not being able to care for my children; I felt guilty for the chocolate chip cookies I had eaten, the glasses of wine I had drunk, the nonorganic chemicals I had used to clean the house. You can't help but go through a phase of blaming yourself. Part of you realizes it's nonsense, ludicrous, insane—but the other part of you plays a tape of your life over and over in your head, looking for a sign or something that could have stopped this from happening.

I also had a few weeks of intense jealousy toward healthy people. Anger came into play throughout, and depression held me for a while. I grieved about losing my breasts and my ovaries, grieved about losing my "old life." Acceptance was slow to come, the slowest of all.

HOLD MY HAND: THE PHYSICALITY OF CANCER

Some people continue physical contact—hugs, hand-holding —throughout treatment, but I didn't want to be touched at all, by anyone. You're not supposed to touch or kiss people, especially kids, for fear of germs. But added to that is your own physical discomfort. For almost a year the only real physical contact I had with people was medical: poking, prodding, sticking, probing, cutting, even monitoring. It began almost immediately when I got the PICC line in my arm; I was constantly watching out for someone to grab my upper arm. I was what you would call hypervigilant. Then my portacath was inserted, so my chest hurt, making hugs less desirable. During chemo there are breaks in the awfulness, when you might feel up to more contact, but after both surgeries I was too sore to be touched. And then radiation burns left me with intense pain in my armpits and chest for almost a month.

Touch is one of the most important senses, and it is an essential part of being human. From the most basic studies on how crucial it is for newborn babies to be held to studies showing that petting an animal boosts mood-boosting hormones, try to maintain some element of touch. Hold a hand—a caregiver's, a nurse's—or pet a dog, cat, or even a rabbit. Many cancer centers have pet programs such as The Pets at Duke Program at Duke Cancer Center in North Carolina. Certified therapy pets visit patients and are there for petting, hugging, and companionship. (There was a therapy dog at my radiation oncologist's office, and his wagging tail was a welcome sight when I arrived for treatment.)

This was an element of my isolation and something I never would have imagined; you just don't realize how much human touch is a part of relating to other people. My head was really the only part of my body I could stand having anyone touch. Then it felt okay to add my feet to the mix. I will never forget the image of my sister rubbing my feet when I was in my hospital room recovering from my surgeries. It was so deeply personal and reassuring.

When my skin healed, I saw an oncology massage therapist in the wellness clinic at my local cancer clinic and she truly changed my life. Getting a therapeutic massage opened the door to getting used to my new self. Ask your medical team if they offer oncology massage services through a wellness program or can refer you to a certified therapist; the treatments are often available for reduced or no cost.

ME, MYSELF, AND I

I was also at one point so sick of me—so sick of everything about cancer and so sick of being sick. I didn't want to talk about it, think about it, or be in Cancerland for one more second. If you're too sick to exercise, work, or even do crafty things like knit or scrapbook, there's a chance you will just wallow. The expression "The idle mind is the devil's playground" came to mind more than once; the more time you have to ruminate, the more you might be tempted to sit and look inward a bit too long. One book I read suggested setting a timer for a daily pity party: ten or twenty minutes allowed each day just to feel sorry for yourself. It seems harsh to me, but it's a good reminder not to spend hours in the bad space in your head. My advice is to see as many movies as possible (comedies and action films only, please—the American Film Institute lists its "100 Funniest American Movies of All Time" at www.afi/100Years/laughs.aspx—make it a goal to watch every single one of them!), enlist funny friends to tell you funny stories, listen to podcasts (there's one for everyone these days), and read stacks of books.

What kept me from dwelling on my own situation was reading about, or hearing about, and eventually meeting, many patients who were so much worse off than I was. It may sound strange, but that motivated me and helped prevent too much self-pity.

You don't control much in this cancer journey, but you can control your mind. Don't forget that. I had a yoga instructor once who told the class that we can do anything for five minutes (this statement was delivered in a pleasant voice as we students balanced on our knees with our arms held out straight in front of us, muscles trembling). That bit of advice got me through natural childbirth twice, and it helped me through parts of my road trip. I won't lie to you; sometimes five minutes feels like five years, and you sit and cry and feel miserable. But I tried to remember that five minutes of what seems unfathomable and impossible will pass.

PSYCHO-ONCOLOGY, OR WHY TO PAY SOMEONE TO LISTEN TO YOU

As a patient, I was also surprised by the lack of comfort I felt at times from family, friends, and medical staff. The things I wanted to talk about: Will I die? How can I handle this completely out-of-control situation? I often felt: I'm terrified and need to share this and no one else will talk to me about it. These were difficult topics for those closest to me to discuss at length. I needed to talk to someone who was removed from my immediate situation. Thankfully there was an oncology social worker at the cancer center who gave me an outlet to talk freely, without having to worry about causing more worry, pain, or guilt to my family. (I didn't realize there was an entire sub-specialty devoted to the psychological aspects of cancer—psycho-oncology—which was pioneered at Memorial Sloan Kettering Hospital in the 1970s.) I also used my therapist as a touchstone: as in, am I crazy or is this feeling/experience/email/conversation completely insane? It was crucial for me to have someone else say, No, no, it's not you. It's cancer!

Don't let finances prevent you from seeking mental health assistance; it is part of your cancer treatment. Also, don't let family or friends stop you from seeking therapy. If you want to go, make the appointment. Many medical centers provide low-cost therapy, and some therapists work on a sliding scale. Some health insurance plans cover mental health; be sure to check your policy. There are many options if you want to see a mental health professional, including oncology social workers, psychotherapists, psychologists, and psychiatrists. (Psychiatrists are medical doctors and are the only mental health professionals that can prescribe medication.) Some larger medical centers, like MD Anderson Cancer Center, have their own dedicated psychiatric oncology departments to support patients. You can also find a national database of psychologists at the American Psychological Association website (www.apa.org).

If professional therapy doesn't appeal, ask your spiritual advisor, priest, or rabbi for some private time to talk, preferably on a weekly basis. I have one survivor friend who relied heavily on her church community, and she still credits them for helping her battle a Stage IV diagnosis while parenting two daughters. Feeling angry with God is a common reaction and something you might want to talk through with your spiritual advisor.

THE MEDICINE CABINET

It's very common to be prescribed antidepressants when you receive a cancer diagnosis—specifically, one or more drugs from a group of selective seratonin reuptake inhibitors (SSRIs), including Celexa (citalopram), Prozac (fluoxetine), Lexapro (escitalopram oxalate), and Zoloft (sertraline). (Generally speaking, SSRIs have fewer side effects than other antidepressants.) Don't feel embarrassed about asking your doctor about an antidepressant. There is a lot of stigma around taking these prescriptions—I've had people say disparaging things to my face—but they helped me when I was so down I couldn't get out of bed. It's something to consider.

Antianxiety medications are also commonly prescribed to oncology patients; Xanax (alprazolam), Valium (diazepam), and Ativan (lorazepam) are the most common. They come in tablet form and can cause drowsiness; discuss any side effects with your doctor. Your oncologist can prescribe these, as can psychiatrists and sometimes general practitioners (also called primary care physicians).

TAKING CARE OF YOUR CARETAKER

Being taken care of is hard, especially when you're an adult. Let's start by saying that at some point during this road trip, your family will lose patience, and might in fact be border-line rude. They will take too long to get you a glass of water from the kitchen—they may even answer their phone on the way!—but you need to let it go. Being angry takes too much energy and precious time. Your family and caretakers are suffering, too—emotionally and sometimes physically. It's hard work to take care of someone you love who looks different and is suffering, possibly even dying.

While you need to focus on your health, you also need to create a little space for your caregiver, even if they won't admit it. They need a break from—let's face it—the grind of cancer care. Whether it's your spouse, partner, family member, or friend, remember a few things to help them stay sane and actually helpful:

- If possible, spread the love. Meaning, rely on a medley of caretakers so one person is not taking on the entire burden of care (which is unsustainable and unrealistic). When your brother tires of getting you lime popsicles at the store across town, ask your best friend. When she's busy, call your cousin to ask her if she can come sit with you. Call Uncle Ed (the one who talks too much and has bad breath) and ask him to drive you to radiation treatment. That neighbor, the one who keeps asking if she can help? Call her and ask her to stay with you until your husband/spouse/partner gets home.

- Say thank you. Not constantly, because you would be saying it about a thousand times per day, but enough to express how much you appreciate their efforts.

- If your spouse/partner needs to take a business trip or travels often for work, encourage them to go. Even if it takes four sets of rotating friends to cover your care, let them bury themselves in work if that's what they need (or want) to do.

- If you're in treatment and dealing with nausea, allergies, or food restrictions, make a list of these and hang it on the refrigerator. That way the food "dos and don'ts" are clear to whoever is popping in to help while your caretaker is on a break.

- Encourage breaks. If you can manage for an hour (or three) alone, send your caretaker off with a smile (and maybe a movie ticket). You will probably want a break, and believe me, they will too. These days, with cell phones, email, and texting, people are usually reachable within a few minutes if there is an emergency. The caretaker might start to feel that they must be there all the time (I heard this from several people), so it might take some gentle nudging to get them to take a rest.

- Remember that there is no one right thing a caretaker can do. They can do a lot of little things, and they will do some things right and some things wrong.

- Don't micromanage. If you like your towels folded one way and Cousin Jenny folds them another, let it go. This is not the time to share your housekeeping tips.

- If you know of a support group or therapist who could help your partner, spouse, or family members, pass on the information to them. If you don't feel comfortable mentioning it, ask a trusted friend to gently do it.

- Caretakers can feel isolated and drained, too. They need time to recharge and reconnect, even if it's in "bits and pieces," as my friend T. said. Small things like getting a haircut or taking a walk are important for the caretaker's state of mind.

- Try to contain (or reserve) any huge bouts of rage that you feel about cancer for your time alone or with your support group or therapist. Try to avoid letting it out over the dinner table or when you're exhausted from treatment. I found it was easy to let cancer rage slip in there when examining the refrigerator and finding there was no more milk or yogurt or some other item that we needed right then, or that the garbage hadn't been taken out, or that the leaky sink hadn't been fixed. Having your caretaker witness said rage is best avoided.

- Your caretaker(s) may qualify for unpaid leave from their job to take care of you under the Family Medical Leave Act. This federal law allows for unpaid, job-protected leave for people meeting certain requirements. See the complete list of criteria at the US Department of Labor website (www.dol.gov/whd/fmla), or have your caretaker ask their workplace human resources department.

OTHER CANCER PATIENTS JUST GET IT: PATIENT SUPPORT GROUPS

While some patients find solace in their friends, family, and spouses or partners, others want to hear from other patients in the same situation. There's something about talking to someone who speaks the same language, who has faced some (or many) of the same challenges and situations you've faced. Patient support groups are usually coordinated through your doctor's office or medical center. Information about groups is often posted on flyers in the elevators and waiting rooms. If you live far from the doctor's office or hospital, connecting online or over the phone with other patients through a nonprofit organization might be an option (see Resources for more information). Many of my survivor friends found groups useful for asking questions and discussing their emotions, treatment side effects, and other topics. However, be prepared for the other side of support groups—that some of the patients in the group won't make it. Besides being heartbreaking and every other word you can think of, that can also be a stressor you might not be up for.

If speaking to people in your situation appeals to you, find out if there's a support group in your area. The more specific the group, the better: You'll have more targeted interactions. Specificity is what makes it so hard to talk about cancer; everyone's experience is different and becomes so personal. But there are enough common experiences that you can hopefully find a group to connect with. A newer support model is a mentor connected by a nonprofit organization; they are trained and vetted and can match survivors with patients. (I think that's a better way to find fellow patients than joining a random Internet forum, but whatever works for you.)

I should say that I never attended a support group. My therapist at the time told me the ones available in my area were for older women and that my needs probably wouldn't be met. (I took that as code for "no one there will really get what you're facing so better to spend your time elsewhere.") And once I began traveling for treatment I just didn't have the time or energy to find another group in my area. But I did ache for one, for a group of people that would just instantly get it, that I didn't have to explain anything to. To belong to a group that would "hear" me appealed on so many levels, particularly the thought that I could speak openly about my health and my life without worrying about whether my kids or my sister's kids were eavesdropping. (Those little ears sometimes hear more than you could ever imagine.)

I did eventually find those people—my people, I call them—but we never met in person. I essentially created my own support group in an unconventional way: I received many kind emails, and a few hospital visits from survivors I had never met before but who knew a friend of a friend. And the bond was instant. They knew what to do and usually what to say to me. I still connect with friends of friends I hear about or "meet" over an email introduction.

PART 2

TREATMENT

CHAPTER 4

CHEMICALS AND CRISPY CRITTERS

There isn't much you can do to physically prepare for chemotherapy, radiation, and surgery except show up at the appointed time. But mental and emotional preparations are a different story. Being aware of the basics can be comforting. The biggest challenge is that once you've finished the first round you know you'll be back in that chair in a few weeks (or whatever cycle you're on). This chapter will discuss what could be coming down the pipeline so you can at least wrap your head around specifics before treatment begins.

Places with Lots of Germs to Avoid While You're in Treatment

- Airplane seatback pockets: Don't touch them!

- Hotel room telephones: Wipe them down with alcohol wipes.

- Indoor kid play areas.

- Steam rooms/hot tubs, particularly public ones, like in gyms, hotels, and spas.

- ATM machines and credit card payment machines: The buttons are crawling with germs; use a tissue or cover the buttons with a piece of paper, or wear gloves.

- Other people's hands: Don't shake hands while in treatment; just smile instead.

CHEMO 101

There is one medical rule of law that no one shares with you when you enter Cancerland: If you can at all avoid it or have any say, never schedule a procedure, an infusion, or really anything at all on a Friday. Getting follow-up care on a weekend is one of the most frustrating things in the world. This goes along with the mantra "be prepared." Compile all the phone numbers of every doctor, assistant, off-hours site, pharmacy, and so forth before Friday afternoon arrives. Murphy's Law reigns in the world of the oncology patient—if something goes wrong, it's usually on a Friday afternoon or over the weekend. (Also, never take the last appointment of the day, no matter what day it is. If the doctor or department is running behind, you could be waiting longer than usual.)

I don't think you will ever really be ready for the first day of chemotherapy. No matter how much you read or hear stories, walking into the infusion center is like the first day at a new school—a completely new environment with its own set of social norms, routines, and smells. Before you begin treatment, your oncologist will ask about exposure to chicken pox and shingles (a.k.a. herpes zoster, caused by the same virus behind chickenpox). If you haven't had either, you might need to get vaccinated. You (as well as everyone in your household) might also be required to get a flu shot.

Chemo is given in cycles for a certain number of weeks, with rest weeks built in so your body can recover. For example, if chemo is administered in week one followed by three weeks of rest, that is considered one (four-week) cycle. But the schedule can vary widely, depending on many, many factors. The amount of chemo you receive is also determined by a number of other factors, including your physical size, the type of cancer, and how advanced it is.

Very generally, the chemo drugs (or agents, in medical-speak) kill cells that divide abnormally. Each type of drug does this in a particular way. Usually more than one type of chemo drug is given (called "combination chemotherapy"). Using a specific combination of drugs can increase efficacy or balance side effects. Depending on the type of cancer, chemo can be given intermittently or continuously. Some types of cancer require a constant ("continuous flow") infusion, delivered by a port that a patient wears at home.

Chemo drugs are divided into seven categories depending on their chemical structure, how they work, and how they interact with other drugs (some drugs fall under more than one group because they act in more than one way).

The main categories of chemo drugs are, in alphabetical order:

- ALKYLATING AGENTS: These work to destroy the DNA of a cancer cell to prevent it from reproducing, and they're used for many types of cancer. The risk with this type of drug is damage to the bone marrow, which increases the risk of developing leukemia, usually five to ten years after use, according to the American Cancer Society. This category is divided into five sub-categories. One of these sub-categories contains what are known as "platin" drugs, which are often grouped with alkylating agents because they kill cells in the same way, but they pose less risk of leukemia. Platin drugs—including cisplatin, carboplatin, and oxaliplatin—are given intravenously and contain a derivative of the metal platinum, hence the name.

- ANTHRACYCLINES: These drugs also alter the DNA of the cancer cells. Long-term use can cause heart damage. This category includes drugs such as epirubicin and doxorubicin (Adriamycin).

- ANTIMETABOLITES: This group of drugs interferes with enzymes to prevent cell reproduction. Cytarabine and methotrexate are examples of antimetabolites.

- ANTITUMOR ANTIBIOTICS: These are not regular antibiotics—they attack the DNA of cancer cells to prevent them from reproducing.

- CORTICOSTEROIDS: Sometimes called simply steroids, these are hormones and hormone-like substances that are considered chemo drugs when used in cancer therapy. This category includes drugs such as prednisone and methylprednisolone (Solu-Medrol).

- MITOTIC INHIBITORS: Used to treat a variety of cancers, these drugs work by preventing enzymes from producing proteins needed for cell reproduction. There are many types, but examples include paclitaxel (Taxol) and ixabepilone (Ixempra).

- TOPOISOMERASE INHIBITORS: These interfere with the enzymes called topoisomerases, which causes the cancer cells to die. Used to treat testicular cancer and leukemia.

- OTHER CHEMO DRUGS: These don't fit into any category because they all act in different ways; one example is the proteasome inhibitor Velcade.

Oncologists recommend chemo for one of three uses: as a cure, as a control, or as a palliative. To be clear, instead of "as a cure," an oncologist might call it "treatment with curative intent," because there is no cure for cancer. When chemo is used as a control, the goal is to control the growth of a tumor—to either stop it from growing or shrink it—including its use as adjuvant therapy (to kill any cancer cells after cancer surgery) or neoadjuvant therapy (before cancer surgery, to shrink a tumor). Or chemo can be used in a palliative way, to keep a patient comfortable in advanced-stage cancer.

The chemo drugs can be administered (or delivered, in medical-speak) to a patient in myriad ways; most often they are given intravenously or orally.

The four most common methods of chemo delivery are:

- Injection (into the muscle or under the skin)
- Oral (in pill, capsule, or liquid form)

- Intravenous (IV; through a vein)
- Intralesionally (injected directly into the tumor)

Other less-common methods are intraperitoneal injection (IP; into the peritoneal cavity); intrathecal injection (into the spinal fluid); intra-arterial injection (into the artery); and topically (on the skin, common for skin cancer treatment).

The First Day

Every cancer treatment facility is different, but there are common elements of the first day of treatment. The area of the medical center or hospital where you receive chemo is called the infusion center. Arrange for someone to drive you there and back; you will not be up for driving, especially as you get further into treatment. You're usually allowed to bring one person with you into the treatment area, but this can vary.

The first stop is the check-in desk. You then might sit in a waiting area until you are walked back to the actual infusion area, where there are chairs (usually vinyl, in shades of blue or green) that, if you're lucky, are the big, comfy versions that can tilt back. If it's a larger medical center or a crowded day, you might be stuck in a plain regular chair. Some centers have several rooms, each of which have a few patients arranged in a circle. Others have chairs lined up along one wall. Some centers have private rooms with chairs or beds. It's usually first-come, first-served, but the sickest patient always has priority.

You'll pass other patients getting chemo: some in hats and pajamas, some in work clothes with full heads of hair—men and women of all ages. (No kids; they are in the pediatric oncology wing.) It's generally quiet except for the beeping of the machines and some quiet chatter. (Bring earplugs if you can't tolerate the sounds.)

The oncology nurse will introduce herself or himself, get you settled in your chair, and then bring over the bags of IV chemo drugs and potentially an anti-nausea drug. Your oncologist should—will, hopefully—stop by to talk to you. The nurse double- and triple-checks your name, date of birth, and the drug order, then hooks you up to the IV either through a vein in your arm or a port (if you have one). The bags are hung up on the metal IV stand and then buttons are pushed on the monitor and the drip begins. Your arm might feel cold as the first bit of IV drug hits the vein, but then you don't feel anything. Some medical centers have warm blankets and even meal service for chemo patients, but otherwise plan to pack a shawl or sweater in case you get cold.

The facility might play a "Welcome to Chemotherapy" video for you, which explains the process and possible side effects in stale, old-fashioned terms. Some survivor friends of mine were required to attend a pre-chemo "prep" class; again, every medical center has its own procedures. You might be required to get blood drawn before the chemo appointment, so allow extra time for that so you're not rushing around.

On your first day, the nurse will monitor you closely to make sure you don't have any immediate reaction (like a rash or other side effect) to a drug. I fortunately didn't have any reaction; I just sat back and tried to read trashy magazines. I never felt like talking—sometimes I watched TV shows on my iPad, but usually I listened to podcasts. Some people knit, read, do crossword puzzles, work on their laptops; some people eat and drink. Depending on the amount of chemo you are receiving and what type of cancer you're being treated for, it can take between one and two hours to complete, although the first day can take up to seven hours while they hydrate you and take extra time to monitor your reaction. (The IV stand is on wheels, so you can roll it to the bathroom with you if necessary.) When the IV stand starts to beep, the infusion is finished. (There is a lot of beeping during chemo; the pump beeps if there is air in the IV line or if the battery is low.) The nurse unplugs you, flushes the IV line with saline, and sends you on your way. You might have to stay in the infusion center for thirty minutes after the treatment is over in case you have any reactions, but again, this varies, so ask the front desk beforehand. The oncology nurses are highly trained and are full of helpful info. You might have the same nurse for every treatment, but they usually rotate.

Your last day of chemo—yes, imagine that!—is also something that will be permanently marked in your mind. On my last day of infusions, a dear friend of mine brought plastic flamingo glasses, and we drank a toast with Martinelli's sparkling apple cider. I have a video of that last beep of the infusion—I don't think I've ever smiled so widely. It still gives me chills when I think about it.

While I did say goodbye to chemo infusions, I continued the oral form of chemotherapy—the trial drug veliparib (ABT-888)—for almost two years after that. Veliparib came in bright green capsules, and I took eight of them every day.

The label on the pharmacy bottles said CHEMOTHERAPY in bold letters and stated that the drug should not be handled, so I wore latex gloves or tried to pour them into my pill holder without touching them. And then I put them in my mouth and swallowed them with water. Daily oral chemo wasn't as debilitating as infusions—my hair didn't fall out and I wasn't throwing up—but I didn't feel amazing. I felt amazed that I was alive, and happy, and lucky. But I often felt nauseous, and exhausted, and not my old self. When Dr. Moasser took me off chemo altogether, after I had been told I might be on it for the rest of my life—it was stunning. My sister and I jumped up and down in the exam room, high-fiving, and pulled Dr. Moasser in for a bear hug. (This is not usual behavior in the cancer care unit, I can assure you.)

Vein or Port?

It's better to receive chemo infusions through a port than through a vein, for several reasons. First, the size of veins can vary greatly: A small vein can be damaged—sometimes permanently—when the chemo enters it, and veins that are damaged or scarred from previous treatment can roll away from the needle, complicating insertion or even slowing the flow of chemo through the body. When chemo hits a large vein, however, it is immediately distributed throughout the body. Second, chemo delivered through a vein can leak from the needle site and cause serious damage to the surrounding skin. The chance of that happening with a port is slim to none. Finally, if you have to receive IV drugs repeatedly, over time veins can start to collapse.

The port also gives you more freedom of movement, especially if you're in the hospital; you don't need to have multiple sites connected to different IVs—everything can be delivered through the port. After the last chemotherapy treatment the port is usually not removed right away; they have to make sure you're finished with chemo, and removal is a surgical procedure that needs to be done by an interventional radiologist or through a scheduled outpatient surgery. Until then, the port needs to be flushed every six weeks by a nurse when it's not in use. (For more on ports, see Cancerspeak, Part 2 in chapter 2.)

The Day after Chemo

On the day after a chemotherapy infusion, you might be required to return to the medical center or office (or sometimes hospitals have outpatient clinics if it's a weekend) to get a shot of Neulasta. This drug is injected into your arm to boost a type of white blood cell called neutrophils. Chemo destroys these cells and can cause neutropenia, a low absolute neutrophil count (ANC) in the blood.

The side effects of the injection can be painful; it can make you feel achy, like when you have the flu. Some doctors recommend taking Claritin, the allergy medicine available over the counter, to help counteract any pain. Nutropin is another blood cell booster given by injection, but that can be administered at home. Neulasta is also available as an at-home injection through the Onpro kit (ask your oncologist).

Household Essentials

You'll discover what you need as treatment goes on, but here's a list of what to keep in the house to get started. I call it the "I've Got Cancer Kit."

- Disposable rubber gloves (Costco sells boxes of them)
- Ginger ale or whatever your go-to beverage is
- A reliable digital thermometer
- Box of individually wrapped alcohol wipes
- Antibiotic cream and Band-Aids in case you get a cut
- Hand soap and hand sanitizer (for you and guests that come to visit)
- Gentle (chemical-free and fragrance-free) body soap
- Disposable face masks (they're not pretty, but if you're sick and/or traveling, you need to protect yourself)
- Soft, cozy socks to wear around the house and in bed
- Mouthwash, breath mints, or lozenges for dry mouth

Chemo Side Effects

The side effects of chemo that can occur are often due to damaged healthy cells in your body. The chemo can't differentiate between cancer cells and healthy cells; it attacks them all. Here are some of the side effects to prepare for:

Hair loss (alopecia): This is common if you're undergoing chemotherapy. Hair starts to fall out slowly, usually after the first or second round. It depends on the type of chemotherapy drugs you're receiving, but it's something to start thinking about. (See Hair: The Bald and the Beautiful in chapter 6 for more on hair loss.)

Urine: Don't be surprised if your urine turns red, orange, or neon yellow during chemo. Some chemo drugs have dye added to them (Adriamycin is bright red, hence the nickname Red Devil, but my sunny friend Dr. K. calls it Red Sunshine). Colored urine can last for up to forty-eight hours after infusion. If after a few days it's still an unusual color or seems bloody or cloudy, tell your doctor. You have to watch for any signs of urinary tract infection, which could lead to a kidney infection. Drink lots of water to help move everything through your system.

Semen and Menstruation: Chemo can affect the smell and color of semen for days and weeks after treatment. Again, drink lots of water and tell your doctor if symptoms seem to last. During chemo, some women experience heavy menstrual flow. This can also happen during radiation for gynecological or colon cancer. However, be sure to tell your doctor about any unusual bleeding or discharge.

Rheumatism: You could experience post-chemo rheumatism, which is pain and stiffness in your joints and muscles caused by the chemo drugs.

Weight gain: Sometimes the chemo drugs cause weight gain. (I gained about twenty pounds during chemo.)

Hormonal changes: Some chemo drugs can cause menopausal symptoms like hot flashes in women. (For more on both hormone therapy and menopause, see Hot Flashes and Mood Swings in chapter 12.)

Eye discomfort: Watery, itchy eyes can develop during chemo.

Bruising: Some types of chemo drugs do strange things to your body. Carboplatin, for example, can lodge in the veins in your arms and darken them after several cycles. I looked down one day and my inner arms were black and blue; they were completely bruised and very sore. It eventually cleared up, but it was just another cancer surprise.

Nails: Chemo drugs can affect fingernails and toenails. Some patients' nails turn yellow or fall out. (For more on nails, see Slap On a Little Lipstick: Small Pick-Me-Ups in chapter 8.)

Neuropathy: Some patients experience extreme neuropathy during chemo or radiation treatment. The most common symptom is a painful tingling in your feet and hands, but sometimes it can be extreme and cause foot problems that need to be discussed with a podiatrist. Neuropathy in the feet can be exacerbated if your job requires a lot of standing or walking. Neuropathy can be very painful, but there are analgesics available, including topical treatments like lidocaine patches that numb the area. Acupuncture is sometimes recommended, as is the nutritional supplement glutamine. Exercise can also ease pain—walking and swimming in particular. These are all options to discuss with your doctor. (See Cancerspeak, Part 2 in chapter 2 for more on neuropathy.)

Temperature: Body temperature changes can also occur. Your body temperature will need to be monitored after chemo. (Invest in a good, reliable thermometer.) Any temperature over 100 degrees Fahrenheit requires a hospital stay, so call your doctor if you develop a fever. Some post-chemo days I felt hot all the time, and other times I had the chills. Just don't be surprised if you are in bed with the windows wide open in the middle of winter while your friends or family are sitting next to you in down coats.

Dehydration: This is a common side effect. It's critical to stay hydrated while undergoing chemo, not only to keep everything moving in your body, but because so many things are affected by dehydration. Constipation and nausea are both intensified by dehydration. That means avoiding caffeine and alcohol; they both contribute to dehydration. (For more on constipation, see page 119.) I drank diluted coconut water as well as tap water with lemon to stay hydrated. Besides over-the-counter medications, the oncologist might prescribe saline or potassium infusions to rehydrate you. I had to sit through six of them—twice a week for three weeks. It's just like chemo infusion, given in a hospital or medical center through an IV, and can take about two hours. I brought books and magazines and had friends visit to pass the time. The drips made me bloated, but other than that there were no side effects (other than boredom).

Other Things to Avoid When You Have Cancer

- Park benches with plaques on them. Most often they're sad. True story: I looked down at a plaque on a bench in our town while I was playing with the kids, and I recognized the name. It was my mom's friend who had died from breast cancer when I was seven years old. It was shocking and haunting and not what I needed to think about in the middle of chemo.

- Obituaries in any form. This includes obituaries in newspapers, alumni magazines, websites, and anywhere else. A lot of people have died of cancer, and you don't need to be reminded of that.

- Hospital settings that don't involve you. Meaning, don't visit people at the hospital or in any medical setting. You have enough visits of your own, and most likely it will just upset you. (And there are germs—lots and lots of germs.)

- Your own head. Don't beat yourself for every "wasted" moment that came before. No one can plan for this.

Nausea: Nausea will become a part of life once you start treatment. The American Cancer Society states that eight out of ten cancer patients experience nausea during treatment. It might be just nausea, or vomiting could make an appearance as well. Certain groups of people have a higher risk of experiencing nausea, and certain types of chemo drugs are known to cause more nausea than others. Be sure to mention any history of nausea to your doctor before chemo begins so you can make a plan together. You do not want to arrive home after your first chemo cycle and have to get on the phone with the doctor or nurse and get to a pharmacy. Plan ahead.

I had a steady level of unbearable nausea thanks to chemo, so I kept a prescription anti-nausea drug with me at all times: in my purse, at my house, and in my car. The nausea was worse during and right after the chemo infusions, and with the pill form it was almost constant. Drugs used to control nausea and vomiting are called antiemetics; a group called 5HT-3 antagonists are the anti-nausea drugs you will get to know. They come in capsule, liquid, and intravenous form. They're usually given right before a chemotherapy infusion or radiation treatment. Be sure to ask your doctor about which drugs are covered by insurance, because some of them are very expensive. You might need pre-approval from your health insurance company, or you may need to coordinate financial assistance to help pay for them. They are an essential part of your treatment, and ultimately, your quality of life.

Common anti-nausea prescription medications include:

- ONDANSETRON (BRAND NAME ZOFRAN): which comes in tablet form and dissolvable (helpful if you can't bear to swallow anything) as well as an infusion and injection. It can be pricey.

- GRANISETRON (KYTRIL): available as an infusion or in tablet form. Sancuso is the transdermal (patch) form; it is expensive.

- PHENERGAN (PROMETHAZINE): available as a tablet, syrup, and injection.

- TIGAN (TRIMETHOBENZAMIDE): available as a capsule or injection.

- COMPAZINE (PROCHLORPERAZINE): available as a tablet, suppository, and injection.

- ALOXI (PALONOSETRON): only available as an injection for severe nausea.

- EMEND (APREPITANT, FOSAPREPITANT): given as an infusion or a tablet. It's a very effective antiemetic but can be expensive. (For me it was more effective as an infusion; I got it as part of my chemo cycle.)

- DOLASETRON (ANZEMET): comes in tablet form; very expensive.

- DECADRON: given as an infusion or as a tablet; it is a type of steroid that is sometimes used to control nausea and stimulate appetite.

For nausea, plain saltine crackers and clear broth are a good start when you literally can't keep anything else down (for more on food, see chapter 5). Trial and error is really the best way to find things that work for you, in terms of both medication and food, so whatever those things are, just stick with them. If apple juice makes the day better for you (and you can keep it down), stock the fridge. If it's one brand of ginger ale, go for it. Some people eat before chemo, some drink juice during it, some eat afterward: There is no "right" way.

If you vomit, have someone look at it and record the amount and color. (My husband had to sift through my vomit to look for the trial drug I had taken, to see if it had been digested! That's love right there.)

Remember, this is a marathon—not a sprint. Just when you think x will happen and you've got this one thing down, something new pops up and y happens. It's part of the patient wait-and-see game to learn how your body reacts to the toxic cocktail you're receiving.

Memory: Another side effect of chemotherapy is memory loss, often referred to as "chemo brain," or more formally as "cognitive dysfunction." Not everyone suffers the same level of memory loss. For me it was cumulative. I would go to brush my teeth, put the toothpaste down, walk out of the bathroom, walk back in, and wonder why I was there to begin with. It was extremely frustrating; it felt like a thick fog I couldn't shake. It also felt like I knew words but couldn't get them out—I would see the object or person in my head but couldn't think of the right word for that particular thing. And memory loss lingered; four months after I was off chemotherapy, I still struggled with certain words and had to write everything down. I carried a notepad and a pen with me always and had someone help me keep my calendar.

This is another reason you need someone (friend or family) to help you, to keep appointments straight, the kids' lives straight. And this is why I bought a seven-day pill holder (the kind with AM and PM slots); it was the only way I could keep track of my medications and be sure I had taken everything in the correct order. Memory loss is a side effect both of chemotherapy drugs and other drugs you might be on. Always talk to your doctor about side effects you experience, but know that you're not alone in wondering, at some point, if you're losing your mind. The good news is that the memory loss eventually fades; it can take longer than you think, but with time your memory comes back. If you experience the fogginess for an extended period of time, ask your doctor; drugs used to treat Alzheimer's patients are sometimes recommended.

Constipation: Constipation is part of being a cancer patient; this cannot be emphasized enough. (Think of it as a nasty gas station bathroom on a road trip; you know it's coming at some point, and you just have to plan ahead.) Many cancer medications, particularly painkillers, will leave you insanely constipated. Opioids, in particular, partially paralyze your stomach and also reduce the urge to defecate, making regular bowel movements difficult. Every single one of my cancer survivor friends mentioned constipation as one of the most frustrating, horrible parts of cancer. And that's saying something.

The medical world has a sexy term for this part of the road trip: bowel management. Your oncologist should prescribe a stool softener and a laxative; Colace and Dulcolax (docusate) are two common brand names of stool softeners, and Senna-Lax (Senna) is a common brand of laxative. They work in tandem, so you need to take them together. One's a softener and one's a pusher, to put it in basic terms. (Powder forms of laxatives, like Metamucil, actually make constipation caused by painkillers worse, according to Harvard Medical School.) Take the laxatives and stool softeners as directed; don't take an extra one to help things along. (Ignoring the dosage instructions can have serious side effects, including interrupting your bowel's natural function.) If the softeners and laxatives aren't working as directed, tell your doctor.

Besides medication, drink lots of liquid. Try prune juice or eating a handful of dried plums; a cup of hot water with lemon can also keep things moving. (Any hot liquid tends to help promote bowel movements.) I tried the herbal "laxative" teas, but they didn't work for me. Last but certainly not least, get moving. Walking or any other form of exercise is crucial to keeping your bowels moving. If you're physically limited, even walking around the house or up and down the street is better than nothing.

Keep in mind that it's much easier to prevent constipation than treat it. My oncologist's quote about constipation: "You have to be aggressive." Besides being uncomfortable, constipation can intensify other symptoms and cause other issues. And really, an enema is not something you want to experience on top of everything else. (This advice to be proactive about constipation might not apply to certain cancer patients, such as rectal or colon cancer patients, so be sure to ask your doctor before taking anything.) If you have not had a bowel movement in three days, call your doctor immediately. Severe constipation may require a hospital visit (besides enemas, digital disimpaction and manual extraction are other ways constipation can be treated).

I would be remiss if I did not mention that you will be talking about poop constantly. Almost every doctor and nurse you meet will ask you whether and when you have pooped and passed gas. It's another benchmark for how your body is reacting to treatment and to the zillions of things you are putting in your body. So get ready for some potty talk.

Big No-No's During Chemotherapy Treatment

- Gardening and yardwork: The risk of infection from cutting yourself and exposing yourself to germs in the dirt is too high. Wear thick gloves or skip the gardening for now (ask a friend to help keep the grass mowed).

- Cleaning the litter box: Cat feces contain a toxin called Toxoplasma gondii that can cause toxoplasmosis and wreak havoc on your body, particularly when you're immune-suppressed. Give the litter box cleaning job to someone else.

- Donating blood: For obvious reasons, you can't donate blood during treatment. (You may be able to donate blood after you've finished treatment; check the FDA policies. Also, each blood center has its own screening protocols.)

- Operating heavy machinery or anything other than a car (and driving might be off the table, too).

- Drinking alcohol in excess. Discuss any alcohol consumption with your doctor, but the bottom line is that alcohol increases the burden on your liver, which is working harder during chemo, and also leads to increased dehydration. Not to mention the fact that you probably won't feel like drinking anything at all because of the chemo.

- Smoking cigarettes, pipes, cigars, and so on. No explanation needed.

Open Wide: Chemo and Your Mouth

Even though chemotherapy is usually infused through your veins, the side effects are felt in your mouth as well. You might experience extra-sensitive gums or dry mouth or develop mouth sores. If you're taking chemo orally, these side effects might also apply.

While you're in treatment you can't go to the dentist; the risk of getting an infection is too great. And after you're finished with treatment, you may have to take a full course of antibiotics every time you visit the dentist. Be sure to ask your oncologist. So you're on your own to maintain dental hygiene.

Here are a few tips to keep in mind:

- Use a soft toothbrush and buy toothpaste for sensitive gums. If you can't tolerate toothpaste, make a paste of baking soda and water. If brushing is just too painful, use a wet paper towel or a damp soft cloth and gently rub it over your teeth and gums.

- Skip the dental floss if your gums are sore or you start to bleed along the gum line.

- If mouth sores develop in your mouth or throat, ask your doctor about a topical anesthetic you can use to help with the pain.

- Rinse your mouth with Biotène Dry Mouth Oral Rinse, a mouthwash specifically for people with dry mouth. They also make a gel for dry mouth; both products are available over the counter.

- If you get dry mouth, keep a pack of lozenges, peppermints, or hard candies in your bag and on the bedside table. Try a humidifier in your room to keep the air moist.

- Avoid eating very dry foods (like hard, crusty bread) and spicy foods; both will irritate the mouth sores.

- Drink as much water as you can to stay hydrated. If your mouth is really painful, use a straw to sip liquids.

- Keep your lips moisturized with lip balm.

Smell You Later:
Why Chemo Makes Everything Smell Terrible

Chemotherapy can change both your taste buds and your sense of smell. While there is no concrete answer as to why, 50 percent of chemo patients report taste changes. Doctors believe they occur because of how the chemo drugs affect the mouth cavity. The medical term for alteration in taste is dysgeusia. (Few doctors give patients a heads-up about this side effect: A 2009 study showed that only 17 percent of patients received information before starting chemo.) Your mouth has one million taste receptor cells, which generate messages to the brain. Different types of chemotherapy drugs (agents) cause different reactions among patients; some types are more likely to cause taste changes than others.

There are no pharmacologic solutions (medication, in other words) for chemo-induced dysgeusia, so it's a trial-and-error sort of thing. I had a constant metallic taste during the first part of my treatment and a bitter taste during the latter part. Ginger chews and dark chocolate took the taste away. Metal silverware might intensify any metallic flavor, so try using plastic forks, spoons, and knives to see if that helps. Just remember, it's not you—it's the chemo. (For more on food, see chapter 5.)

To keep smells to a minimum, cover drinks with lids or drink through a straw. Also try to eat (or just hang out) in a room with an open window or other source of fresh air. If you're bothered by strong laundry detergent, perfume, or other strong scents, ask your friends to post a sign by the door so friends and family can go fragrance-free on the days they visit you. (You could also post this request on your social media outlets if you have a page for friends and family; for more on social media, see Journals, Emails, Blogs, and Other Public Airings in chapter 1.)

SURGERY

Some types and stages of cancer are treated with surgery, so whether you're lucky enough to skip chemo entirely or you're done with chemo and cleared for surgery, this is the section for you. As I've mentioned before, the word "surgery" may be mentioned and the possibility discussed with your medical team, but you may find yourself forgetting the details of what will happen and what you will feel like afterward, once the initial conversation is over. I had two separate surgeries about a year apart, and this is what I can pass on to you to make the whole experience a bit smoother.

Surgery Prep

Whether you're going in for colon cancer surgery, oral cancer surgery, or a mastectomy, there are myriad elements involved in preparing for the big day. (Bigger surgeries, such as amputations, are not covered here.) A pre-surgical meeting is scheduled with your surgeon or surgeons in their office to go over the procedure and the possible risks, and to answer any questions you may have. Depending on the type of surgery, your surgeon may bring up tissue donation (skin, bone, organs, or blood). Some medical centers have a tissue bank and use tissue for research. It's entirely anonymous, although certain information like your age, race, and gender are needed.

After meeting with your surgeon, you might attend a surgery prep class at the hospital three to four weeks before surgery. (Again, every hospital and medical center is different. Some require a class and some don't even offer them.) These prep classes are usually two-hour sessions run by surgical nurses who review general questions and hospital procedures, like what time to check in to the hospital and the types of anesthesia, as well as answer any questions you have. (Every patient in the class is there for a different surgery; in my class, one woman was going in for a knee replacement, another was getting foot surgery, and so on.) I brought my sister with me to take notes and keep me company. I was absolutely terrified of surgery, and that isn't something that is generally addressed by doctors. Surgeons are justifiably confident in their abilities, but what is an everyday, routine job for them might be a once-in-a-lifetime (hopefully) experience for you, so fear and terror are normal emotions for patients. (The technical term is "pre-surgery anxiety.") I found talking through the procedure and getting more information from reliable sources (in other words, not the Internet) helped me calm down. Alternative methods of coping with fear such as guided imagery and affirmations are being used more and more in medical centers. The mind-body connection, as it's referred to, is getting more attention from the medical community. I practiced some visualization techniques; there are numerous "preparing for surgery" audio books available at bookstores and through iTunes and Audible.com. Ask your medical team if there are any pre-surgical patient workshops available that address fear and anxiety. I also had a list of "surgical affirmations" that I read over and over. I also threw in some prayers; the more the merrier when it comes to preparing your mind for surgery.

Next, a nurse from the hospital will call you before the surgery to go over specific information such as allergies, medicines, and what type of surgery you're scheduled for (yes, it's the left breast and not the right, or it's the left kidney and not the liver). They will confirm your arrival time at the hospital (generally early morning for a major surgery). Remember to request early morning if you have any input at all. A hospital surgical schedule is just like a flight schedule: As the morning goes on, there are more delays that can occur, and the last thing you want is a postponed surgery. As with most medical appointments, try to schedule surgery early in the week (this depends entirely on the surgeon's schedule, but you can try). The medical team will also advise you to stop smoking and stop drinking alcohol thirty days before surgery; this helps reduce the risk of infection.

Finally, the day (or night, as I experienced) before your surgery, the surgeon will call you at home to check up on you. You will be instructed to wash your body from the neck down with antibacterial soap the night before surgery. They will confirm that you aren't eating or drinking anything after a certain time, or that you're taking a certain medication if required. In my case, the gynecological oncology surgeon who was removing my ovaries "reminded" me to take an oral laxative. No one had told me this bit of news before, so my husband had to hightail it to a twenty-four-hour pharmacy to pick up some, and I guzzled it down in one gulp. Needless to say, it wasn't an ideal scenario the night before surgery. So be sure to ask questions about any medications, procedures, or anything else you're wondering about, and then ask them again. (Despite that little hiccup, I came through my thirteen-hour surgery without a hitch!)

Remember: You cannot eat or drink anything for twelve hours before surgery! (It's called the pre-surgery fast.) Don't sneak a handful of M&M's or a sandwich and then plan to lie about it in the morning. It's a serious hazard—you could vomit under anesthesia, which could lead to infection, pneumonia, and other complications. The surgery could also be canceled if the surgeons are aware of any liquid or solids in your body, so just stick to the rules and do the fast.

The last, most important bit of advice: Confirm the location of your surgery! Some medical centers have more than one location, and there's always a chance you might mix up the addresses. Have a loved one/caregiver/friend triple-check the address, check-in time, and parking situation, if applicable, to make the surgery day less stressful than it already is.

The Big Day

Almost every major surgery is scheduled for the early morning. (The actual surgery might be scheduled for 10:00 AM, but you have to arrive two or three hours before that.) Did I mention I was nervous before both of my surgeries? My mom stayed with our kids and my husband, and I slept at a friend's house near the hospital, then my husband and I drove in silence in the dark morning to the hospital. (I was trying to stay calm and didn't want to talk.)

We parked (surgical patients get priority parking), then headed to the check-in desk. And here is a play-by-play: Flash your photo ID (sometimes two forms of ID are required), sign the admissions paperwork, get a hospital ID wristband, and head to the surgical wing. One or two family members (maximum) can be with you; it's nice to bring someone who is calm or can crack jokes.

The hospital is remarkably busy for that time of day; lots of rubber-soled shoes squeaking and a sea of people in colored scrubs. The admitting nurse brings you to a hospital room where you change into a hospital gown and put your clothes in a plastic bag. You cannot wear anything after this point, including contact lenses, jewelry, and hearing aids. Your family can hold your things, or the hospital will provide a storage locker (I will never forget handing my wedding rings to my sister to wear while I was in surgery).

Then you climb into a hospital gurney (essentially a bed on wheels) and start the anesthesia process. Various nurses and doctors may ask you the same questions repeatedly; this is part of the triple-check system. You are handed a blue paper surgical "shower cap" and get prepped for an IV. You will meet the anesthesiologist, and your surgeon(s) might come by. (For plastic surgery, the surgeon will come by with a permanent marker and mark the areas that he or she will be working on.) At some point you will be handed a clipboard and an informed consent form to sign. The nurse chats as he or she starts to hook up the "sleepy drugs," and you begin to feel groggy. Kiss your family goodbye, and you're wheeled down the hallway into the operating room. My last vision was the surgical team and a big silver light. And then I woke up.

Tumor Registry

No, it's not as fun as a wedding registry, but a tumor registry could ultimately save you and other cancer patients. This is a national database that collects data from patients, including details like age, race, and size of the tumor. (There is no data that identifies you as an individual, such as your name or address.) Each state tries to track every case of cancer and reports this data to the national database. This helps doctors discover whether there is one type of cancer that's more prevalent in one area of the country and can help determine if there are larger factors that are causing those types of cancer in certain populations or areas. The Centers for Disease Control and Prevention (CDC) runs the National Program of Cancer Registries (NPCR); they also work with the National Cancer Institute (NCI) Surveillance, Epidemiology, and End Results (SEER) Program.

Post-Op and Recovery

Everyone experiences pain differently, but there are a few things to expect after major surgery.

You will wake up in the recovery room. I wasn't prepared for how groggy I would feel or the fact that I would be barely conscious (I could only move my eyes and whisper a few words for the first few hours). Usually the hospital allows two family members to visit very briefly, and only one at a time.

After a few hours you are moved to a hospital room. (There are fewer restrictions on visitors once you're out of recovery.) I was lucky enough to get a private room; ask the nurse when you check in that morning if one is available (put that on someone else's to-do list).

Your throat might feel sore from the breathing tube that was inserted in your mouth while under anesthesia. You most likely will feel pain in the surgical area, and you might have bruising and swelling there, too. (After my double mastectomy and salpingo-oophorectomy, I felt like I had been hit by a bus.)

Depending on the surgery, any sutures are usually left in for one to two weeks and will be covered in bandages. Only the doctors or nurses should touch the bandages; leave them alone! The goal is to prevent any infection.

The hospital will give you their own list of suggested items to pack, but this is what I found helpful during my hospital stays:

- Photos of my family (I propped them up on the windowsill or taped them to a wall where I could see them from the bed).

- Photos of my "calm place," such as the mountains, a beach, or a vacation photo.

- Pillow and cotton pillowcase.

- No-elastic socks or slippers.

- A cozy blanket or scarf to use as a wrap.

- Bottled water.

- Essential oils like lavender and rosemary mixed with water in a little spray bottle. I asked my sister to spritz my hospital bed—the aromas soothed me and took away some of the hospital smells.

- No-rinse face wipes to clean your face.

- Baby powder or cornstarch (to sprinkle under your arms or wherever you need a little freshening). You won't be showering at the hospital.

- Body or hand lotion (your skin will get dry).

- A hat or scarf for your head (in case you get cold).

- Glasses, if you wear them (you won't be able to put in or take out contact lenses).

- Electronic tablet, e-reader, or portable DVD player (hospital televisions are usually terrible) and any electronic chargers.

- A cell phone with charger (you probably won't feel up to calling anyone, but you can receive texts, and friends and family can use it to call).

- A friend or family member.

The best things in my hospital room were my family and friends. They took shifts sitting with me, and it made me feel less helpless and alone. You might not be able to watch TV because of the all the meds (they can make you lose focus), so load up a device with podcasts, or bring audio books and a CD player (cell phones and similar devices aren't permitted in some areas). My friend Barbara sat with me and read out loud until I fell asleep. It was so comforting.

You are required to wear a hospital gown while at the hospital, so don't bother packing any cute pajamas.

While you're in the hospital make sure you verbalize your needs! If you're in pain, speak up. If you need water, say something. (And get your family or friend to help you vocalize.) If you are ignored, keep asking. I had to ask (actually, make a strong suggestion to) my doctor for an additional night in the hospital after my double mastectomy and salpingo-oophorectomy because I didn't feel strong enough to return home after one night. (Some surgeries may require long hospital stays; be sure to discuss this ahead of time with your medical team so you're not caught unaware. See the sidebar below for more about preparing for longer stays.)

A Room at the "Inn": Preparing for Long Hospital Stays

Use these steps to prepare and plan for treatment or surgery, such as a bone marrow transplant, that will require a significant hospital stay (more than a week).

- First, find out exactly how many days you will be admitted to the hospital as a patient. Some larger medical centers have housing for patients after a pre-op treatment but before they are actually admitted as a patient. Often this housing is in the medical center itself, and sometimes it's free of charge.

- Ask about "life" details like laundry and meals. Sometimes rooms have small refrigerators, but you often have to bring your laundry to a Laundromat.

- If the hospital doesn't have housing and you live more than a few hours away, there are many foundations that can help. Try not to add a long commute to your already-stressful situation. If you know people in the area, you might also ask friends and family if anyone has an extra room you can stay in.

- If you are a caregiver who needs to stay with the patient in their hospital room, ask about cots, sleeper beds, or sleeper chairs and shower/bathroom facilities for you.

- Ask about "sitters," who will stay with a patient while the caregiver gets a break. Again, larger hospitals often have sitters on staff. Particularly if your caregiver is staying round-the-clock, he or she will need a break.

- There is a patient white board in every hospital room that lists the doctor's name, the name of the charge nurse, emergency numbers, and other information the nurse writes down with an erasable marker, including goals for the day, which I always found amusing (the goals could be "walking unassisted down the hall," or simply "standing up"). Be sure your caretaker and any other friends write their phone numbers on the board in case of emergency.

- Remember, during a longer hospital stay your caretaker needs breaks—a walk outside, some decent coffee, something besides sitting in the hospital room for twelve hours a day. As my friend T. said as she took care of her husband who had brain cancer, people came to the hospital to keep her company. Often her husband wasn't even aware that she was there, and she needed friendly faces and support.

Returning Home

Planning for your return home is a critical step. Depending on your surgery and your housing situation, you might need to make adjustments such as having someone help you up steps or move a bed into the living room.

Be sure you and your caregiver are both clear on post-surgical "dos and don'ts." For example, mastectomy patients cannot use ice packs or heating pads on the surgical area. Check the surgical area for bruising or swelling; a certain amount is expected, but you need to call the surgeon if something seems amiss.

The second consideration is follow-up appointments. Make sure you, a family member, or friend takes detailed notes about the days and times of post-surgical appointments. If you have to see more than one doctor, book the appointments on the same day, especially if you live more than a few miles away from the hospital or doctor's office. The big thing you will be waiting for is the pathology report ("path" for short), which will show how much cancer was removed. It's usually available within a week of surgery.

When you're discharged, the nurse will review your list of medications. Be sure these are filled at the pharmacy before you get home. Getting home can be painful, depending on your surgery, and you want to be able to get into bed and take any prescribed medication immediately so you can start healing. Hospitals almost always have pharmacies, and your prescriptions can be filled while you're signing discharge paperwork and getting discharge instructions.

The drive home is the first step. If you've had chest or neck surgery, make sure you have a large pillow with you to put between you and the seat belt. For other surgeries, you might need a pillow under your legs or rear end. Be sure to ask the nurses ahead of time so you can give your family or friends a list of what you will need. This list might change if you are taking a taxi home; note that most hospitals will not allow you to take a taxi home alone. There must be someone to accompany you home after surgery.

If mobility is a serious issue, you might need to rent a wheelchair, cane, or walker from a local medical equipment supply store. This should all be ready for you when you arrive home. You won't have the energy to arrange those accommodations on your first day out of the hospital. The drive home in and of itself is completely exhausting.

Bathroom trips may require new accommodations. If you can't access your toilet or bathroom, a rental toilet chair can be helpful (horrible to think about, but in fact very handy). The official medical term for this type of equipment is "durable medical equipment" (in case you see the phrase on forms, charts, or health insurance claims).

For most surgeries with sutures, you won't be able to shower by yourself or get the incision area wet for two days. (A hand-held shower attachment is very helpful.)

If you have drains inserted (officially called Jackson-Pratt, or JP, drains) after a mastectomy, they need to be emptied, with the liquid measured and recorded for the surgeon (they can often tell if something is wrong if there is too little or too much discharge) two to three times per day. This is a job for someone with a strong stomach (the fluid is usually bloody and yellow), so unless your loved ones are up for the job, consider hiring a nurse or home health aide. Also, you cannot drive until after the drains are removed.

If you have wounds that require dressing or bandage changes, you will need to arrange for someone to do that. (The hospital should send you home with the necessary supplies; be sure to ask the nurses at the hospital.) Following a single or double mastectomy, you won't be able to move your arms without pain for at least a few days or lift anything heavier than a gallon of milk for six weeks. Following a mastectomy, men's cotton undershirts are the best thing to wear while recovering. The armholes make them easy to put on and allow access to the drains; they're soft, easy to wear under a wrap or robe, and they're inexpensive, so you can throw them out when your breasts have healed!

If possible, rent a hospital bed. My surgeon didn't mention it, but other patients did and it was the best thing in the world. I could move it up and down and get out of it much more easily than my regular bed. (This is especially true if you sleep on a low or platform bed.) You also might want to invest in a set of inexpensive cotton bed sheets. Depending on the type of surgery, you may have blood, sweat, or other fluids that can stain the sheets. We put absorbent cotton sheet covers—available at medical supply stores and some pharmacies—to protect the mattress under the sheets. It's worth the investment; you won't want to look at those sheets once you've healed. Again, these are the things that make a big difference in quality of life, but they might be out-of-pocket expenses, so it's important to plan ahead.

You might have to rearrange a room or the house or apartment to accommodate your recovery. If you live in a space with stairs, you might have to convert another room into the bedroom. (I had to recover for a few days right after surgery at my sister's house, where there was a bedroom and bath with no stairs in between.) I also needed a space where I could walk around a bit without using any stairs. Moving around, even for a few minutes a day, is crucial to prevent constipation, and having a safe space to walk around is critical.

Another small thing that made a huge difference in my recovery was moving a TV into the bedroom. For the first two days it was so nice to be in bed and just zone out and watch something, or have friends sit and watch with me when I didn't feel up to talking.

Recovery time from surgery varies. Most people return to work three to six weeks after breast surgery, but it obviously depends on your diagnosis and the type of surgery you've had. Ask your oncologist if physical or occupational therapy would assist your recovery.

My wise sister had a helpful timeline to share from the caretaker perspective: Day one is usually fine for patient and caretaker because you are still on the meds from the hospital. Day two is so-so; the meds start to wear off and your body is adjusting to its new state. Day three is "hump day"; you feel the worst as the trauma of the surgery hits and the anesthesia has worn off. The good news is that it usually only gets better from that point. The most important thing to remember is that everyone feels what they feel and literally every body is different. The doctor will say, "You should feel x or y" by a certain day, but you need to say how *you* feel. You know your body better than anyone. Again, don't be afraid to speak up.

Unveiling

One of the hardest moments in the entire cancer road trip was the day I went to get my bandages off after my double mastectomy. The emotions are so complicated. I was so eager to get my breasts removed—they represented illness to me—but to look down at my chest that day left me in shock and tears. (And I can't say the nurse was terribly helpful; she took one look at my face and told me she'd give me a minute, and left the room.) My husband was with me, and my dad was on a stool behind the curtain. I was just devastated. I just cried. My advice: Don't go alone. Have someone you trust more than anyone in the world there with you while your new body is revealed.

On the flip side, some women are excited and delighted at the unveiling and don't shed a tear. Be prepared for a wide range of emotions.

Breast Reconstruction

If you're a breast cancer patient who has chosen breast reconstruction, you will be meeting with a plastic surgeon for what should be a one-day surgery, or at most will require an overnight hospital stay. In 2014, more than 100,000 breast cancer patients had reconstruction after mastectomy, according to the American Society of Plastic Surgeons.

A few facts to consider while you're making a decision about implants: You can still get a mammogram with breast implants—there is no additional risk of recurrence associated with implants—and you can get reconstruction after mastectomy or lumpectomy. (Check the NCI website for the most recent research and statistics about reconstruction.)

You don't necessarily have to make the choice immediately. Talk to your doctor about the timeline. Some women can have immediate reconstruction, which means the breast implants are inserted during the mastectomy or lumpectomy surgery, while others have to wait until they complete other treatment such as radiation (radiation changes your skin, so the plastic surgeon needs to stretch the skin beforehand so it can expand and make room for the implant). If you are scheduled for delayed reconstruction, the plastic surgeon will insert tissue expanders that act as placeholders for the actual implants. The expanders are filled up, week by week, with saline injections in the surgeon's office. It's essentially like a balloon that is being inflated. I'm not going to lie: It is not a comfortable process to have a needle stuck into your breast(s) while you're wide awake (there is no anesthetic). It feels tight across your chest on the day it's filled, and some weeks it was just unbelievably uncomfortable for days afterward. (Ask someone to drive you to and from these appointments, if possible.)

Alternatives to Breast Reconstruction

If you've decided that breast reconstruction isn't for you, consider a breast prosthesis (also called a breast form). It's a breast-shaped insert made from silicone gel, foam, or fiber-fill. There are three types: partial, shell, and full, and each can come with a nipple or without. You can get a premade or a custom form, which is created by taking a mold of your chest wall. Some breast forms are weighted, and you can choose adhesive forms (which use a special glue to stick to your skin if you want to go braless) or magnetic forms (which use magnets to adhere, and for which you have to carry a card to show airport security—you will set off the metal detectors!).

Prosthetic bathing suits are also available if you're worried about hitting the beach or the pool after mastectomy. Breast forms can also be fitted and sewn into any bra; you just need someone who sews and who can be sure it is fitted properly. You generally have to wait six weeks after surgery before using any type of prosthesis. If you're receiving radiation therapy, be sure to wait until after treatment and after your skin has completely healed before choosing a prosthesis; your skin—as well as your sensitivity—in the chest area can change. (Health insurance often covers the cost of breast prostheses; see Resources for more information.)

Here's the basic process if you're prepping for reconstruction. Before the surgery date you will meet with your "plastics" person (that's shorthand for plastic surgeon) and, in what may be the most surreal moment of the whole road trip, they will hand you two blobs that look like skinless, boneless chicken breasts—these are the two choices for your new "ta-tas": saline or silicone. (I chose saline, for what it's worth.) Both types of implants require a new "set" about every ten years, which is an outpatient procedure. Generally you choose the cup size, although that can depend on your bust size before surgery. You can bring in photos to help show what your ideal pair would look like. Another tip I heard from a few doctors and nurses: Always go smaller than you think. Final tip: Do not go online to look at any photos of breast reconstruction—some of them are frightening. Get your information from fellow patients and your surgeon.

Here are some pros and cons of the two types of implant options, but keep in mind that the most important part of reconstruction is finding an experienced plastic surgeon:

- SALINE IMPLANTS: silicone shells filled with sterile saline (saltwater) solution. Saline implants are inserted empty and then filled with saline through a needle in the doctor's office. If an implant leaks, it will deflate and the saline is simply absorbed into the body. The shell must then be surgically removed.

- SILICONE IMPLANTS: silicone shells filled with silicone gel. Silicone is a plastic, and silicone implants are said to feel more like natural breasts. They are inserted into the chest pre-filled. If an implant leaks, the plastic surgeon will have to remove the implant surgically. Often there are "silent leaks," or undetected leakage that can have side effects. The FDA recommends that patients with silicone implants get periodic MRI scans to check for silent leaks.

With both types of implants you might need to change or restrict certain forms of exercise, so be sure to ask the surgeon. With some exceptions, you can breastfeed with breast implants.

Depending on the type of breast cancer you have, your nipples might be removed as well. Plastic surgeons refer to the surgery as nipple-sparing or skin-sparing, or non-nipple- or non-skin-sparing. If your nipples are removed, the surgeon can "build" nipples and areolas out of skin, or you can get both nipples and areolas tattooed on your skin by a tattoo artist who uses special pigmentation (there are tattoo artists that work with surgeons and hospitals). Either way, you won't have any feeling in the nipples because they are no longer connected to the nerves in your body. Or you can just go without them altogether.

You might need additional skin for the reconstruction. Sometimes surgeons can take skin from one area of your body and move it to the breast area. But often they use a layer of AlloDerm, which is cadaver, or donor, skin that has had the cells removed, leaving only the collagen. It is placed under your skin, like laying the foundation of a house, so you can't feel or notice any difference. Ask your surgeon about the pros and cons of the different procedures.

Be sure to ask your health insurance company about what is covered for breast reconstruction. Ask about pre-surgical visits, the surgery itself, and post-op visits. Some health insurance companies require a second opinion before they will approve the procedure.

Scarface (Or in My Case, Scarchest)

Scars from surgery or procedures like port insertions are often part of survivorship. There are two main types of post-surgical scars: keloid and hypertrophic. Normally scars go from thick and red to thin and white in about sixteen to eighteen months. There is no way to surgically remove scars, but there are a few ways to minimize them. There is just no way to know how much they will fade. (The appearance of scars also changes if the surgical area is exposed during radiation treatment.) Over-the-counter creams are an affordable solution. Products like Mederma, as well as natural oils like almond and coconut oil, are options. With most topical creams, it might be at least thirty days before you notice a difference. If you're scheduled for radiation therapy, be sure to ask your radiation oncologist before you use any topical cream. Some creams and topical ointments can interfere with treatment. Dermatologists can be consulted for scar treatment, including prescribing certain creams, but the office visits and treatment might not be covered by your health insurance plan.

Some side effects from scars can surface years after surgery, as a result of something like pregnancy or significant weight gain (especially if your surgery was in the abdominal area). If you notice any changes in the scar, call your surgeon.

RADIATION 101

Radiation therapy is a common treatment for cancer and is performed by a specialist called a radiation oncologist, who uses a linear accelerator to send proton beams to destroy the tumor and cancer cells inside your body. Fortunately, radiation therapy has come a long way since the first beams were aimed; while it's more targeted and safer than ever, radiation can still have potentially serious side effects. In addition, there is only one chance with radiation; you cannot radiate the same part of the body more than once per cycle. The bottom line with radiation is essentially a cost-benefit analysis: Is it worth the risk? This is the conversation you will have with your radiation oncologist.

Radiation therapy is broken up into doses, or treatments, that can range from days to weeks, depending on the type of cancer and severity. Each treatment is done in an outpatient setting—it does not require a hospital stay. Radiation therapy is usually done after—or in some cases, instead of—surgery, because it can affect the skin.

There are two main types of radiation therapy:

- External beam radiation (usually delivered through the linear accelerator machine)
- Internal radiation therapy (or brachytherapy)

If you've decided to move ahead with radiation, your treatment plan will be formulated by the radiation oncologist and a specialist called a dosimetrist. They use computer programs to calculate the amount of radiation needed to shrink the tumor while considering any possible damage to surrounding tissue. The amount of radiation is measured in a unit called a Gray (Gy) but can also be measured in centigrays (cGy), which is one-hundredth of a Gray. (This is a very simplistic explanation of a very complicated procedure, but at least you get the idea.)

Then, often a cast or mold is made of the treatment area. It's molded out of plastic and is an exact replica of your body position that you will be in during therapy. (My position was lying down on my back holding my arm above my head in a sort of crescent moon shape.) The last planning day involves a lot of marking of the skin (they used to tattoo tiny dots to mark the target areas, but most cancer centers now use permanent marker), taking photographs, and making adjustments to be sure the beam is going exactly where it's intended to go. The radiation oncology team might also set up foam blocks or forms to place over other parts of your body to protect them from the radiation. You might also have a bolus (a piece of malleable plastic) placed over the treatment area, which allows the beams to go even deeper into the tissue below without damaging the external skin. If you're receiving radiation on your head or neck area you will probably wear a mesh head mask, which prevents your head from moving during treatments.

Radiation therapy involves lying down on a table with a large machine very close to your body, so it will definitely test your patience, your muscles, and any claustrophobia tendencies you may have. (If you're really feeling agitated, talk to your doctor about meditation, visualization, or prescription medication options before each appointment.)

Before radiation appointments begin, the radiation oncologist will give you a printout of your treatment field, which is the area to be radiated. The more areas being radiated, the more fields you have. The first color printout of my "fields" was a crazy mess of white lines and looked like something from a modern art museum.

A typical appointment involves checking in, changing into a cloth gown and pants (depending on the area of treatment), and sitting in a waiting room until the radiation tech calls your name. You cannot wear any lotion, deodorant, perfume, or creams; they can interfere with the treatment.

You will likely have daily appointments at a set time, and the office is almost always running on time (in other words, no waiting!). Tardiness is not tolerated! Be sure to arrive on time; there is so much that goes into the setup of a radiation therapy appointment that patients need to be prompt. The actual treatment session takes only about one to five minutes (depending on the dose), but with the setup the full appointment can be thirty to sixty minutes. (There are some forms of radiation treatment that are administered twice a day to accelerate the process.) Each week the radiation oncologist will take X-rays to confirm that the radiation is hitting the intended area.

The radiation oncology techs work with the radiation oncologists and are the ones who actually operate the linear accelerator machine; you won't see the doctor for every single appointment. The radiation oncology nurse will work with you to coordinate treatment and can address any concerns. I relied on my nurse so much—she was amazing, kind, and always available to me by phone or email. And the techs are the best; they position you in the machine, then they might put music on for you (many medical centers have music libraries of CDs; I usually plugged my iPod into the speaker system), and they basically become your "radiation buddies" for the duration of treatment. It can be a fairly intimate thing, depending on where you're getting radiated, so you get comfortable with each other pretty quickly.

Before I began radiation, I was completely clueless about the process. My most memorable radiation moment happened on my first day of treatment. I walked in and asked if I could put on sunblock (I get freckles and a sunburn with the tiniest bit of sun). And the radiation oncologist, nurse, and staff looked at me like I had three heads. "No," they said. Because the point is you need to burn to get to the cancer cells. Little did I know!

Although radiation therapy is targeted to a specific area, it will affect surrounding tissue when the beams go in and out of your body. You don't feel anything right away—any side effects build up over time. In my case, burn wounds developed about thirty days in.

Burns are generally the most common side effect. External burns are like any other burn to the skin and usually start with small blisters or a bad sunburn. With internal cancers, like throat or tongue cancer, the inside of the mouth (including the tongue) and the throat can become severely affected. (Chef and oral cancer survivor Grant Achatz wrote extensively about this in his incredible book *Life, on the Line.*) It's something to prepare for when planning meals; you might need to drink only liquids and shakes for a period of time. Internal long-term side effects are something to discuss with the radiation oncologist. A good friend of mine who had radiation for colon cancer was warned about damage to her bladder as well as vaginal tightening and dryness—things that might seem unimaginable. I was warned of potential damage to my heart, given that my treatment field encompassed the left side of my chest. Another friend with non-Hodgkin's lymphoma was warned of damage to her throat. That's another odd, surreal moment of the road trip: You are warned about these side effects, but there is literally nothing you can do other than forego the treatment entirely. You simply add the line "monitor side effects" to your survivorship list.

Other external radiation therapy side effects include fatigue and itchy skin. Fatigue does not mean just being tired; it's being tired regardless of how much sleep you might get. (For more on sleep, see chapter 7.) It usually builds up over the course of treatment. Itchy skin is something else to watch for. I was so itchy by the third week of treatment I had to wear rubber gloves so I wouldn't tear my skin when I scratched.

If you have surgery before radiation and any nerves are involved, nerve pain can also increase with radiation therapy. (Gabapentin is a commonly prescribed medication for nerve pain; ask your doctor.)

Before Each Treatment: Skin Prep

If you're receiving external radiation (rather than internal for colon cancer or oral cancer, for example), preparing your skin before each treatment session is crucial for long-term recovery. Radiation oncologists usually have their preferred skin treatment, but there are many options and remedies. If something doesn't work, try another product. And remember to talk to your doctor about your prep routine.

Here are some commonly recommended products:

- LANOLIN (or wool fat) is an emollient, meaning it creates a layer of oil on top of the skin to trap moisture and prevent flaky, dry skin. (It's available over the counter.) The flip side of all the moisture, however, is that the skin can get too moist and a yeast infection can develop. Signs of a yeast infection include red skin and itchy, small white bumps. Tell your doctor immediately so they can treat it promptly; I got one and it was not pleasant. I saw yet another doctor—a dermatologist—and got yet another prescription filled. Note: If you have a wool allergy you most likely will not be able to use lanolin, so talk to your doctor.

- ALOE VERA, in gel form, can be applied both before and after radiation treatment and is available over the counter at any drugstore or health food store. Just be sure it is alcohol-free; alcohol is very drying to the skin. (I kept a bottle of aloe vera in the refrigerator so it was cold and even more soothing when I applied it.)

- One percent HYDROCORTISONE CREAM can be used as a topical remedy to treat any burning (available over the counter), but ask your doctor before using it. A stronger (higher percentage) version is available by prescription if needed.

- CALENDULA CREAM is a vegetable or lanolin-based topical cream that is infused with calendula flowers, known for wound-healing properties. It's available over the counter at any drugstore or health food store.

- SILVADENE (silver sulfadiazine) is a prescription-only topical cream used for treating radiation burns.

- RADIAGUARD (lidocaine) is a topical cream available over the counter intended to help skin heal and regenerate after radiation.

- BIAFINE is a topical cream, officially a "wound dressing," made in France. It works by adding moisture to help the skin heal and protect the wound from contamination; it leaves a slightly waxy residue on your skin after application. While it used to be a prescription-only cream, it's now available over the counter at drugstores and online at Amazon.com. Be sure to tell your doctor if you're using it during radiation; you cannot apply it within four hours of starting radiation treatment.

- AQUAPHOR is a fragrance-free topical cream available over the counter. Hydrophor is a similar product—it's a topical ointment that contains mineral oil and lanolin.

- MEDIHONEY is a topical cream from Australia made with honey. I smeared it on some red areas that developed, and it was effective; it's thick and sticky but has a pleasant aroma. (It's available through your radiation oncologist.)

- Some radiation oncologists recommend sprinkling pure CORNSTARCH over the radiated area before and after radiation therapy. The cornstarch absorbs moisture. This is particularly true if you're getting radiation in the folds of your skin (armpit, neck, groin, and similar places) or wherever you feel sticky or sweaty (especially if you're getting treated in the summer). Apply it with a clean makeup brush for easy dusting over your skin.

Note: All of the creams can stain or ruin your clothes! Buy five or six loose, inexpensive, 100 percent cotton T-shirts before treatment and wear those. And keep them on at bedtime to protect your sheets and bedding.

Here are some other tips for taking care of your radiated skin:

- Watch your skin for any changes and tell your doctor. I got deep burns inside my left armpit that had to be treated, which interrupted my therapy; it's imperative to tell your doctor immediately if you see any changes.

- If you see any bubbles or blisters develop on the skin, do not touch them! Tell your doctor immediately, and they can recommend a cream and a dressing.

- Use warm water instead of hot water in the shower to avoid irritating your skin.

- Use very gentle, fragrance-free soap in the shower.

- If you are getting radiation on your breasts, wear a non-underwire bra after treatment. Some doctors recommend going braless—a cotton camisole is a perfect alternative.

- If you're feeling very itchy, place an electric fan on low and let the air blow over the radiated area. It can help soothe the itch and discomfort (especially in warmer climates or months).

- Stay out of the sun! Cover the radiated area completely for one year after the last day of treatment. (My radiation oncologist told me that if left uncovered and unprotected from the sun for the first year after treatment, any skin reaction I had during treatment could become permanent.) Wear a hat, a scarf, and long pants and shirts—whatever blocks the sun. This is in addition to applying sunscreen with an SPF of 15 or higher on your non-radiated skin areas. Sun-protective clothing with a UPF (ultraviolet protection factor) of 50+ is also a smart way to protect radiated skin (available at sporting goods stores or online). See Resources.

- Avoid chlorine, which is extremely drying and can exacerbate any skin reaction. If you must be near chlorine, try covering the radiated area with a layer of petroleum jelly before exposure.

- Avoid any hot areas, such as steam rooms and saunas. (You'll probably start to feel warm from the radiation and want to stay as cool as possible, anyway.)

- Don't soak radiated skin in water, such as hot tubs or baths.

- If you're getting in the car when your radiated skin is feeling particularly painful and sensitive, you might want to put a cotton pillow or small blanket over your chest before you put on the seat belt.

PAIN

Pain is often part of this road trip. Pain can be caused by the cancer itself (a tumor pressing on nerves, joints, bones, or organs), by tissue destroyed from cancer, or by the treatment. Regardless of the source, you should not suffer through pain. (According to the Mayo Clinic, one in three cancer patients undergoing treatment experiences pain.)

The goal is maintaining a quality of life as you go through treatment. Pain is a stressor—it stresses both the mind and body, so don't ignore or diminish it. Don't be shy about expressing your pain to your doctor; seeking relief does not label you as an addict.

Most pre-appointment intakes include the question, "Are you in pain today?" The medical world uses a scale of 0 to 10, 0 being no pain and 10 being the worst pain. They will ask you this over and over and over again. If you do have pain, you need to describe it: Stabbing? Tingling? Localized? In one arm? Or one foot?

Pain is broken down into two types:

- ACUTE: Begins suddenly, has a clear source, and doesn't last long. Can also increase heart rate and blood pressure. (An example of acute pain is stubbing your toe or burning your hand on a hot pan.) This type of pain is part of the "fight-or-flight" response; it's a warning signal to stop doing that activity in order to survive.

- CHRONIC: Can come and go and last a month or years; can affect mood and appetite, and has little or no effect on blood pressure. There may or may not be an obvious source for this type of pain. This is the most common pain that cancer patients experience.

If your doctor is not responsive to your questions about pain relief or doesn't seem to have enough information, ask for a referral for a pain specialist. (I consulted one for my nerve pain, and it completely changed my quality of life.)

There is a wide range of pain relief available. The medical term for painkillers is analgesics. From over-the-counter relief to prescription-based, highly regulated drugs, there are pain relief options. (Certain painkillers require the patient to present a written prescription and state ID or driver's license at the pharmacy, and sometimes you—rather than a friend or family member—must pick them up in person. Just ask ahead of time and plan accordingly.) Also, while most pain relief is given orally, there are also rectal, IV, or skin patches available if you can't swallow a capsule. If you're concerned about side effects, talk to your doctor; it might take some trial and error to get the right dosage, but the proper dosage should relieve pain and not leave you completely "out of it."

What were once considered alternative options such as acupuncture or massage are now considered complementary therapies in some medical circles. (Some of these options are offered through medical centers, and in some cases through health insurance satellite centers.) Considering every option, both traditional and nontraditional, is critical to finding the right pain relief.

Here are some basics on your options, from alternative to mainstream:

- ACUPUNCTURE: Some patients find pain relief from acupuncture (an element of Chinese medicine that involves inserting needles into certain points on the body). But be sure to ask your doctor beforehand; some doctors advise against it due to concerns about infection, and clinical trial protocols may prohibit it.

- MASSAGE: Some patients find massage relieves pain. However, be sure the massage therapist is familiar with therapeutic massage techniques, particularly if you are at risk for developing, or have, lymphedema—incorrect massage techniques could cause fluid buildup. Some medical centers offer therapeutic massage or can refer you to a reputable massage therapist.

- MEDITATION AND HYPNOTHERAPY: Some patients find relief through what some call the mind-body connection. Working with a licensed hypnotherapist or using self-hypnotic techniques might be worth considering. (The American Society for Clinical Hypnosis is responsible for licensing in the United States and is a good source for finding a clinical hypnotherapist.)

- TOPICAL PAIN RELIEF: For muscle, joint, or bone aches a topical pain reliever might work. I use Sub Zero, a topical pain-relieving gel that you rub directly on your skin. It provides some relief and goes on clear.

- OVER-THE-COUNTER (OTC) PAIN RELIEVERS SUCH AS IBUPROFEN (ADVIL, MOTRIN), ASPIRIN, AND ACET-AMINOPHEN (TYLENOL): These mild pain relievers can sometimes have more severe side effects in cancer patients, so talk to your oncologist before taking any of them. A prescription dose of acetaminophen (called Q-Pap) might be prescribed. Again, be sure to tell your oncologist before taking these during chemo because they increase the risk of bleeding if your platelet count is low.

- MILD OPIOIDS: These include prescription medications like codeine.

- STRONG OPIOIDS (A.K.A. NARCOTICS): Strong opioids are prescription medications like hydromorphone (Dilaudid), oxycodone (OxyContin, Percocet), morphine (Avinza); methadone (Dolophine, Methadose), oxymorphone (Opana), and hydrocodone (Vicodin).

- NERVE BLOCK: For severe pain, the doctor might suggest a nerve block, which is an anesthetic injected near or into a nerve.

CLINICAL TRIALS:
TO BE A GUINEA PIG OR NOT?

Clinical trials are research studies on people. When I first heard the phrase "clinical trial," I shook my head, stomped my foot, and said no one was testing a thing on me. The word "experimental" can strike fear in a patient; after all, who wants to be the first person in line for a potentially life-threatening treatment? But without clinical trials, medical research—particularly oncology—would be at a standstill. Clinical trials allow a drug manufacturer to prove the efficacy of a new drug or treatment before it can be prescribed by a physician (or before it "goes to market"). Trials go on all over the world, and they need human volunteers—patients, called participants or subjects. One example of just how important trials are to medicine is evident in the standard treatment for breast cancer. In 1970, the only viable treatment was the radical mastectomy. Since many clinical trials have shown other options to be just as effective (less-invasive surgery, radiation therapy, and less-intensive chemotherapy regimens), breast cancer patients now have many more treatment options. I had to switch my thinking from viewing clinical trials as exposing me to "life-threatening" experimental drugs to seeing the drugs as "potentially life-saving."

Clinical trials are many-years-in-the-making sorts of things, and they are monitored very closely. The trials are overseen by the FDA and run by the drug company (called a drug sponsor) through medical centers. There are strict protocols; ignore the mythical image of a bunch of mad scientists looking for a few willing volunteers. It takes an average of twelve years for a drug to go from discovery to FDA approval, and ninety percent of drugs in trials fail to get approval. A lot of thought, effort, and research goes into the drugs that do make it to the trial stage.

Another myth I had to overcome was that clinical trial participants are always facing a last option; there are trials for every stage and every type of cancer. At the same time, you, the patient, have to qualify for the trial—they don't accept every patient that comes along. It's an interesting juxtaposition; the drug company needs you and you might need them, but it's a delicate dance. Factors such as the type and stage of your cancer as well as your age, gender, race, and prior treatment (if any) are considered before you are admitted, because every trial is very specific. It's often a complicated process to find, and enter, a clinical trial.

Finally, you must remember that you are volunteering to participate. You can decide to leave the trial at any time.

Here's a very basic summary to help explain what exactly goes on in clinical trials. First, there are three types: The first is a treatment trial, which evaluates a new type of treatment (surgery, drug, radiation therapy) or a combination of treatments to see if they are better than the treatments currently available to cancer patients. The second is a quality-of-life (also called supportive care) trial, which studies ways to improve the quality of life of cancer patients and survivors who have gone through cancer treatment. (The goal with this type of trial is not necessarily to cure or slow the growth of disease.) The third type includes prevention, diagnostic, and screening trials. These trials study ways to lower the risk of getting cancer. The participants in these trials vary widely; some might not show symptoms of disease; some have had cancer and are at risk of recurrence or have developed a cancer other than the original diagnosis. The trial is overseen by a doctor from the drug manufacturer who works with the clinical trial doctor at the specific location where the trial is taking place. Every hospital or medical center participating in the trial follows the same rules and guidelines (called the protocol).

There are four phases of a clinical trial—Phases I through IV—and each one has a different focus. These phases occur in all three types of trials. In every phase the doctors monitor the safety and side effects.

Before Phase I begins, the drug company applies to the FDA to begin a clinical trial based on preclinical research. Once they receive approval, they can move to:

Phase I: This phase is based on a set of preclinical trials or research and involves a small number of patients (twenty to forty). Phase I determines the best dose and delivery method (intravenous versus oral) of a drug and how often the drug is given (called the schedule). This phase can take several months, up to one year.

Phase II: This phase involves a larger group of patients and usually focuses on the effectiveness of the drug against a specific type of cancer. Phase II also usually involves twenty to forty patients (although larger Phase II trials can have one to two hundred patients), and it can take up to two years.

Phase III: This phase examines the risk-benefit analysis of the drug or combination of drugs being tested. For cancer drug trials, the medical team studies the safety and efficacy and compares the new drug against the current standard of care for a particular type of cancer. This involves a large number of patients, sometimes thousands, usually a variety of gender, race, age, and other factors to show the wide use of the drug; it can take years to complete. When the results of this phase show that it helps patients (or "leads to better outcomes" in medical-speak), the drug manufacturer submits the findings to the FDA. They review the results and determine whether the drug is allowed to be "released to market," or available to patients (prescribed by physicians) for a specific use.

Phase IV: Sometimes a drug or drug combination requires further study, or a Phase IV, which involves studying the long-term side effects over a larger group of patients.

Even after the drug is released to market, the drug sponsor is required to provide ongoing safety data to the FDA. (Side effects are recorded and released to doctors and public health officials; if the side effects become severe, the drug can be pulled from the market.)

Finding a Clinical Trial

Clinical trials are listed in online databases that can be accessed by both doctors and patients. While your doctor may have other ways to find trials, particularly if they are part of or connected

to research hospitals, you and your support system can start by
researching trials on these well-regarded websites:

- The Center for Information and Study
  on Clinical Research Participation:
  www.ciscrp.org/our-programs/search-clinical-trials

- CenterWatch: www.centerwatch.com

- City of Hope: www.cityofhope.org/clinical-trials

- Coalition of Cancer Cooperative Groups:
  www.cancertrialshelp.org

- National Cancer Institute: www.cancer.gov/about-cancer/
  treatment/clinical-trials/search

- National Institutes of Health: www.clinicaltrials.gov

- Patient Resource:
  www.PatientResource.com/Search_Clinical_Trials.aspx

Here are a few clinical trial terms to know:

- PLACEBO: A placebo is an inactive substance that is given
  to patients in a clinical trial; it's given in the same way
  and looks the same as the trial therapy. It is intended to
  mimic the therapy. ("Placebo-controlled" means a trial in
  which the control group is given the placebo.)

- RANDOMIZED OR RANDOMIZED CONTROLLED TRIAL
  (RCT): An RCT is a trial in which patients are randomly
  assigned one of two treatments: the control (a placebo or
  no treatment at all) or the actual treatment. This allows
  the two groups to be compared equally and objectively.

- DOUBLE-BLIND: Some trials are conducted on a double-
  blind basis, which means neither the doctors nor the

participants know which group they're in (meaning which type of drug, or placebo if applicable, they are taking). This helps protect the results from any influence from the researchers or participants.

There are clinical trials happening all around the United States, every day of the week, every week of the year. But finding and enrolling in one requires research. It's not as easy as it sounds. Finding an open trial that might work for your particular cancer takes perseverance.

If you or your doctor have found a trial that could benefit you, there are questions to ask before you sign on the dotted line. Before you enroll in a trial, make a list of questions for the trial doctor. Remember, the trial will most likely not be run by your oncologist (who may be able to explain only the basic details), so you will meet the trial doctor to discuss the details of the trial.

Here are a few sample questions to get started:

- Is this a randomized trial?

- Is it a placebo or non-placebo trial?

- How long will the trial last?

- How will the doctor determine whether the treatment is working?

- What kinds of procedures (such as infusions or surgeries) are involved in the trial?

- What (if any) are the results of previous studies of this particular drug or treatment?

- What will the follow-up be?

- Where is the trial? (Sometimes the trial is only available at select hospitals. Travel reimbursement is often not provided, so you have to ask ahead of time and take the psychological and financial burdens of traveling into consideration.)

- Are there any medications that would prevent me from participating? (Sometimes the trials are open only to patients who have not received certain drug therapies or medications; be sure to ask.)

The Cost of Participating in a Clinical Trial

Even though you're volunteering for a trial—you're receiving the drug and treatment free of charge—there are still costs associated with participating. Under the Affordable Care Act (ACA), all insurance companies must cover the routine costs from an in-network provider associated with an approved clinical trial. (An approved trial is defined as one in any phase that is aimed at treating, detecting, or preventing cancer, and is either federally funded or federally approved. There is a bit more fine print; ask your health insurance company to review the trial to be sure it's covered. And individual states may have further requirements, so you might have to do some serious digging.) Unapproved, or experimental, trials are a whole other topic that you need to talk to your oncologist about.

If you're uninsured, set up a meeting with the hospital or medical center's patient financial services department promptly. They can often help with certain costs or find resources from a hospital foundation or grant. Don't let finances stop you from exploring this option if the trial is recommended by your oncologist. The American Society of Clinical Oncology, or ASCO, has a patient website—www.cancer.net—that offers detailed information about clinical trials.

What to Expect in a Clinical Drug Trial

If you've found, and decided to enroll in, a clinical drug trial, an entirely new part of the road trip begins. (Think *detour* with a capital *D*.) Most likely you'll be at another hospital or medical center. But the most startling thing about it is you'll become a number rather than a person. In February 2013, I became Subject Number 985.

A trial by definition has to be blind, so the only identifiers are numbers: your subject number and test results. For me it was particularly striking because I worked so hard to define myself as a person as well as a patient—and suddenly I was just a number. Being a number was frightening to me; it strips you of any personal markers and makes you anonymous. Some days in the hospital I just wanted to scream and shout, "Look at me! I'm a person!"

You, the patient, give written, informed consent—you've been informed about the treatment and potential risks and you agree to proceed—when you enroll, but always remember that you can leave the trial at any time. Keeping that in your back pocket is essential to remembering that you still have a say. Yes, you're lucky to be in the trial, but feeling lucky doesn't factor in to your overarching emotion. I didn't feel lucky on the days I had to suffer a twelve-hour fast followed by a four-hour infusion, all while spending two days away from my daughter and son. Ultimately, you still have a voice.

The other surprise to me was how isolating a trial can feel. Often you won't meet any other patients in the trial (I never met one single person). There are no message boards, support groups, or weekly meetings. It's surreal; you're all part of this one club, but everyone enters through a different door at different times. So if you are looking for a communal experience, a trial probably won't satisfy that need.

Clinical Trials by the Numbers

Reprinted from "Patient Resource Guide to Understanding Clinical Trials, 2nd edition," Patient Resource Publishing, 2015.

- 10: Number of cancer-related drugs approved in 2014

- 85: Percentage of clinical trial drugs that face delays because of a lack of qualified and interested participants

- 73,155: Number of clinical trials registered in the United States as of April 16, 2015

- 20 to 40: Percentage of patients eligible to participate in clinical research

- 2: Percentage of patients ages 20 to 39 who are participating in clinical trials

- 5: Percentage of women with gynecologic cancers who participate in a clinical trial

- More than 300: New medications that have been approved by the FDA over the past ten years; about 97 percent of them are still on the market today.

CHAPTER 5
FOOD

Road trip food can be iffy, and it's exactly the same during cancer treatment. My life before cancer revolved around food. If you're anything like me, and the thousands of other foodies out there, you can relate. I'm a trained chef, I've edited cookbooks and helped other people write their own, and I grew up with a mom who cooked every single night and threw dinner parties every weekend. I'm the type of girl who finishes breakfast and then thinks about lunch, and dinner, and possibly breakfast the next day. (Throw two kids and a husband into the mix and we've got a lot of food lists.) I would drive twenty miles for the perfect baguette or get up at 7 AM to grab the best croissant in town. The only "diet" I've ever been on was the doctor-prescribed, no-raw-cheese-sushi-cold-cuts-or-alcohol regimen for pregnant women. If no one lays down the law, however, I'm in for raw, deep-fried, truffled, and flambéed. Champagne? Pour me a glass.

So it comes as something of a horror when eating becomes a necessity instead of a source of pleasure. You may stop cooking entirely. I did. I didn't have the energy or the interest. And cooking bland food depressed me. What was the point?

Taste buds change with chemo drugs, and mouth sores often develop; suddenly you're down to about five things you can stand to eat (or look at) each day. For me it was noodles, beef, pizza, toast, and yogurt. And when a chef friend came to visit, I found a sixth food group: Korean barbecue! (The moral of that story: Close no food doors.) Throw in the smell factor (see Smell You Later in chapter 4 for more on how chemo affects your sense of smell and taste) and it's no wonder food becomes a bit of a thing.

Of course, you can't expect everyone to know your cancer food cravings. And when people find out you have cancer, they assume you need sugar and they start to bake. A spoonful of sugar makes the medicine go down? Cookies, brownies, bars, and cakes will appear in droves.

And though it's more of a food additive than a food, the other "treat" people drop off with uncanny regularity is marijuana: buds, lollipops, and brownies. Or maybe this is just a California thing. At one point I had enough marijuana to get the entire town stoned. (See the sidebar later in this chapter for more on medical marijuana; it can be an option to stimulate your appetite and provide pain relief.)

There was one way I incorporated some of my old foodie life into part of my cancer routine. I knew exactly which sandwich at my local bakery I could stomach before or after treatment, and on my trips to Los Angeles for my clinical drug trial treatment I always tried to research new restaurants I could try with whoever came with me. My *Los Angeles* magazine was circled and dog-eared as we made our way to the "best cookie in the valley" or the "best sandwich in Glendale." We always stopped for salads and bread at a bakery in Pasadena, and the staff remembered me every time. It made me feel as if I had more people cheering for me. These adventures made the trips more bearable: less medical and more magical thinking. We could pretend—if just for one meal—that we were on a vacation, down in Duarte, California, for no other reason than for the sheer pleasure of it.

My favorite cancer food memory is when my husband brought Lebanese food to the hospital after I was allowed to break my ten- to twelve-hour fasts during the early days of the drug trial. He walked in with two huge bags of food, and the young nurse in my room just stood there, wide-eyed, as he opened container after container: hummus, tabbouleh, kebabs, pickled radishes, pita. All my favorites were there, and I was ravenous. I started shoving food into my mouth. Then I looked at her and said, "Is this okay?" And she said, with no humor in her voice, "Yes, except if your stomach explodes." I rolled my eyes and kept eating.

EAT, DRINK . . . YOU HAVE CANCER

People—friends and perfect strangers—will start to ask you what you're eating. If I had a dollar for every time someone asked me if I was "still eating meat." Everyone has a theory about food and cancer and they all want to share it with you. People will tell you how this vitamin helped them, or how they avoided dairy, or ate the fruit of a rare plant. (Often the advice simply comes in the form of the food itself: "healthful" soups, tofu stews, or raw beet salads are delivered with great gusto.) These food comments will usually be shared with a bit of a superior tone and a sad shake of the head if you admit that you've eaten half a pepperoni pizza and a popsicle that day. If you tell people what you're eating they might comment; just be prepared.

WEIGHT WATCHERS

Connected to food by a straight line is, of course, weight. In Cancerland, weight maintenance and weight gain are usually the goals, unless you've come to cancer extremely overweight. Why? Because fat equals energy. You're going to need some energy to get up every day, breathe, and make it to your appointments. And your body needs all the energy it can get to fight off those lurking cancer cells.

In most hospitals, an oncology appointment begins with the weigh-in. Remove your shoes and any heavy jewelry, and wait for the beep of the electronic scale. I think of it as a perverted version of Weight Watchers. Instead of points for an ever-dropping number on the scale, you get points for keeping weight on. (This is a tricky topic, however: Some people gain weight from chemo and others lose weight. There's no rhyme or reason.)

The doctors have list upon list of foods you should be eating to stay healthy and hale—think lean turkey sandwiches rather than cheeseburgers. But there are two kinds of foods that doctors might instruct you *not* to eat: The first is grapefruit—whole or juiced. Grapefruit contains furanocoumarins, which block an enzyme that normally breaks down certain medications in the body. When the enzyme is left unchecked, medication levels can grow toxic in the body. (Other citrus fruits like Seville oranges, limes, and pomelos also contain furanocoumarins, but the drug interaction isn't as well-studied.) This usually only applies to medication taken orally, but ask your doctor to be sure. The second is antioxidants—chocolate, tea, blueberries, and so forth—because you need to keep all the chemo in you and antioxidants help eliminate "bad" things from the body, which isn't the goal during treatment. And ask your doctor before taking any vitamins, minerals, or supplements during treatment. There are some severe drug interactions with certain vitamins, so don't swallow anything unless you've cleared it with the docs.

But here's the thing: You're already taking their pills and doing everything else they tell you to do. Do you really have to take their advice on food, too? Except for the grapefruit and antioxidants, I ate what I craved, and nothing anyone told me about vitamins and health and bone recovery would make me eat barley soup when all I wanted was pizza. (Man cannot survive on pizza alone, but if it's a choice between no food and pizza, choose pizza.) Make that call for yourself, but know you won't be alone when you "just say no" to cauliflower-parsnip soup!

During one chemo cycle I was eating the only things I could stomach—mouthfuls of bread, rice, broth, and water—to no avail; I still lost two pounds that week. When I finally had my first real meal after that round of chemo (spaghetti and meatballs!), I felt like throwing a parade.

But, of course, the wrinkle with weight gain and eating what you want is nausea. (For more on nausea, see Chemo Side Effects in chapter 4.) Being turned off by food is depressing for most; it'll drive the desire to eat right out of you. For those moments when you must eat (and you really must eat; don't add malnutrition to the list of ailments) but would rather do just about anything else, here are some recommendations, which come with the unofficial stamp of approval from a large sampling of my cancer-survivor friends:

- Stock the freezer with popsicles. They are a no-brainer when you have mouth sores, and they're good just for general ease of eating (plus you can always share them with the kids). And these days there are all sorts of flavors, including somewhat healthy beet-and-carrot popsicles that taste a bit like cherries. Ice cream works, too, although dairy can be iffy on your post-chemo stomach.

- Locate the nearest 7-Eleven, then head to the Slurpee section and order a big one.

- Lemonade and limeade: The citrus does something to drive away the nausea.

- Gingersnaps were my favorite cancer cookie. Ginger in any form—ginger ale, ginger tea, ginger chews—can help with nausea. But I most loved soft, slightly chewy gingersnaps. (For a recipe for ginger cookies that kept me going through treatment and beyond, see the sidebar later in this chapter.)

- Smoothies: If you can't stand the thought of a steak—or even a pat of butter—but are short on necessary proteins, try a smoothie. Start with a fruity base like a banana or frozen strawberries (or whatever is appealing), and add protein powder, peanut butter, almond milk, or whatever protein you need to get through the day. (You can also add a handful of spinach for some greens; you won't even taste it.) There are also pre-made shake blends that just require ice. If you're really desperate and on the road, order a milkshake from the nearest restaurant.

- Rice: When you can't face "real" food, a big batch of fluffy rice is one of the easiest things to get down. (Rice is particularly helpful if you're seeing friends or eating out but can't imagine stomaching anything real. Almost every cuisine on the planet involves rice of some sort, so it's easy to find.)

You will find most doctors reluctant to suggest any specific foods to eat that are "cancer fighting." Most often my doctors told me just to eat what I could keep down. Although I was forbidden to take vitamins during treatment, my sister did a little research on foods that might boost red and white blood cell counts. I was so desperate to keep them up so I could continue to receive chemo (low counts can lead to being kicked out of the clinical trial) that I probably would have eaten bugs if offered. But cooking certain foods that might boost my "counts" did give me (and my family) some sense of control; whether it worked or not is up for debate. I tried eating fried or sautéed oysters to boost my white blood cell counts, and beef bone marrow soup or fresh bone marrow on toast for my red blood cell count. (And frankly, sometimes I wanted to eat those things anyway, so it wasn't a burden.)

Medical Marijuana

Medical marijuana (or cannabis) is often in the headlines, but few people really know much about it. There is a difference between the psychoactive (recreational) drug and medical marijuana. There are two main ingredients in the plant: the cannabidiol (CBD) and tetrahydrocannabinol (THC). If the CBD levels are higher than the THC levels, the plant is less psychoactive. Research has shown that medical marijuana is an effective treatment against a variety of medical issues, including glaucoma, multiple sclerosis (MS), the wasting syndrome from HIV/AIDS, and chemotherapy side effects such as vomiting and nausea.

Medical marijuana is something to consider if other painkillers or antiemetics aren't working, but it's important to keep your doctor in the loop in case of any drug interaction or clinical trial drug protocol rules. (As of this writing, twenty-three U.S. states and the District of Columbia have legalized medical marijuana.) There is one form of medical marijuana that requires a prescription from a medical doctor and can be purchased at a traditional pharmacy. Called Marinol or dronabinol, it's a form of marijuana with the THC removed; it comes in capsule form, and you take it like any other oral medication. Side effects include sleepiness, vertigo, and appetite stimulation.

Nausea can intensify if your stomach is empty. A few of my survivor friends would eat every two hours to keep the nausea at bay. Again, it's trial and error. (For more on nausea, see Chemo Side Effects in chapter 4.) Though ginger teas and "energizing" herbal concoctions were often given to me by well-meaning friends, they never did the job. They're still stacked up in my cupboard like a leaning tower of Pisa.

On that point, if people are dropping off meals and asking you what you like and dislike, tell them. And let nausea be your guide, as you might be nauseous more often than not during chemo and radiation (and post-surgery). I asked for not-too-spicy foods, no creamy soups, and no fish—those were a few things I couldn't face during chemo. Other cancer friends outlawed meat, broccoli, and anything red. Friends and family want to make something you will eat, so don't worry about hurting anyone's feelings by saying you want jars of strawberry jam or baked manicotti. And never say "no, thank you" to someone who wants to bring food. Whatever you can't eat now, you can freeze for later . . . or you can serve it to your family. I had amazing, resourceful friends who sent gift certificates to local take-out restaurants and food via the Internet; everything from bread to ice cream was delivered to my door. Finding delicious food waiting on my doorstep was exactly the kind of help I needed, even a year into my illness.

If well-meaning friends are all used up or thousands of miles away and you still need food assistance, ask your doctor or treatment center if local meal services are available. There are many organizations that will deliver food to cancer patients; when you can't get to the store, these are a godsend (see Resources for more information).

If you're really in a food rut—taste- and nutrition-wise—ask your doctor about a nutritionist or dietician. Almost every cancer center has an on-staff nutritionist or dietician that will meet with you to discuss food and diet. (They can help you before, during, and after treatment.)

The Most Delicious Ginger Cookies in the World

No, that's not what they're actually called, but these are the cookies I ate over and over (and over) again while in treatment. The best thing about them is that anyone can make them; they are literally foolproof. My foodie friend (and cookbook author) Kurt Dammeier graciously allowed me to reprint the recipe.

GINGER CRINKLES

Makes 36 cookies

2¹/₄ cups all-purpose flour

¹/₄ teaspoon table salt

2 teaspoons baking soda

2 teaspoons ground cinnamon

1¹/₂ teaspoons ground ginger

¹/₂ teaspoon ground cloves

1 large egg

¹/₂ cup neutral-flavored cooking oil, such as canola or soybean

3 tablespoons unsalted butter, melted

¹/₄ cup plus 1¹/₂ tablespoons blackstrap molasses (see Note)

1 cup packed light brown sugar

¹/₂ cup granulated sugar

1. Preheat the oven to 375 degrees F.

2. In a large bowl, sift together the flour, salt, baking soda, cinnamon, ginger, and cloves.

3. Using a handheld mixer or stand mixer fitted with the flat beater attachment, mix together the egg, oil, butter, molasses, and brown sugar at medium speed, scraping the bowl once or twice while mixing. Add the dry ingredients to the mixing bowl. Mix at low speed to incorporate the flour. Scrape the bowl once or twice while mixing. Stop mixing as soon as the dough is uniform.

4. Place the granulated sugar in a shallow medium bowl. Form the dough into 1^{1}/$_{2}$-inch balls and roll 4 to 6 balls at a time in the sugar until each ball is completely covered in sugar. Place the balls 2 inches apart on an ungreased baking sheet.

5. Bake the cookies for 8 to 10 minutes for a chewy cookie. For a crisper cookie, bake for 12 minutes. Cool the cookies on the baking sheet for 5 minutes before carefully transferring them to a cooling rack to cool completely.

Note: Blackstrap molasses makes the cookies darker and gives them a richer flavor than regular molasses. It is also full of vitamins and minerals, making it more nutritious than many other sweeteners. You can find blackstrap molasses at most grocery stores, but you can substitute light or dark molasses if you prefer.

Make ahead: The cookies will keep in an airtight container at room temperature for up to 5 days.

Reprinted with permission from *Pure Flavor: 125 Fresh All-American Recipes from the Pacific Northwest* by Kurt Beecher Dammeier with Laura Holmes Haddad; Clarkson Potter/Crown Publishing Group, 2007. All rights reserved.

CHAPTER 6

FALLOUT

You can lose a lot of things along the cancer road trip: your hair, your energy, and even your fertility. This chapter discusses some ways you can cope with some of what I call the Fallout.

HAIR: THE BALD AND THE BEAUTIFUL

Watching your hair fall out in chunks onto a pillow is scarier than anything you can imagine (even if you're not a hair prima donna). The doctors warn you it will fall out, and then the waiting begins. Will it happen a few days after the first treatment? A week? Two weeks? Will I wake up one morning completely bald, or will it be a slow, consistent shedding like an animal losing its winter coat?

What I was unprepared for was seeing the chunks and then wisps of hair that would float down to the floor every time I moved. I didn't realize hair sticks to flannel sheets like Velcro. I lifted two fingers to scratch an itch on my scalp and a fistful of hair came out. At that point I was one chemo treatment in, and that fistful was pushing me over the edge.

It was disturbing—and what disturbed me most was how much it upset me. Before then I had thought, who needs hair? I made little jokes about being liberated from the hair dryer. But when the day actually came and the hair started to fill the bed, the hallway, and the bathroom, I felt like I was in a horror movie.

There was only one option, in my mind: I would get my head shaved. I had a romantic notion of driving to the city to see a hair stylist who closed her salon once a month for cancer patients (a worthy cause if you can find a salon in your area; see Resources). I thought: a head shaving, a little shopping, a little lunch. But when I called she was booked for a week. And I couldn't wait a week; I could barely sit up for ten minutes without wanting to throw up. So we drove five minutes to a local hair salon my mom used to go to, with hairdressers who had known me since I was ten. It seemed rather cosmically aligned, to be somewhere familiar while something so unfamiliar was happening to me.

I called ahead and told the receptionist I wanted my head shaved. Confused, he said, "I'm sorry?" And I replied, "I have cancer and need to shave my head." Two hours later I sat down in a chair in the window and tried not to cry as the stylist fastened the black smock around my neck. My sister was with me, and another survivor friend too, and they held my hand and took pictures while I tried not to look. It took about fifteen minutes and a few different blades to become bald. My white head looked shocking in the lights and mirrors of the salon. It's surreal to go from a face you've seen a million times in the mirror to seeing a stranger. "You have a nice head!" my friend said, patting my shoulder. I rubbed my hand over my head, feeling the ridges of my skull—smooth but a little stubbly—and tried to smile. We had brought a silk scarf along, and my sister placed it over my head and pulled it in a chic knot. We walked across the street and she bought me a pair of large, Audrey Hepburn–style sunglasses and then we went out for cheeseburgers.

Eventually the rest of your hair (yes, that hair) will go, too, like you're a molting bird. I lost all my hair except my eyebrows and my arm hair. It's startling how startling it is. But you get used to it. The shock wears off, and one day you realize your mornings are pretty snappy without hair: a two-minute shower, throw on a scarf or hat, and you're out the door.

Besides scarves, hats and wigs are other options. Most medical centers have baskets of cotton and wool knit hats made by survivors or donated by local volunteers, which are great to wear in the winter. I had a little black cashmere cap I wore in January and February and often even in bed. (I never knew how cold your head gets without hair!) Bandanas are also good—I know a few male cancer patients who went that route, but since bald is "in" right now, no one really notices when a guy loses his hair. To keep my dome nice and shiny (and moisturized), I rubbed pure coconut oil on it every night (olive, grapeseed, jojoba, and almond oil will also work). If oil feels too greasy, try a facial moisturizer or a light, unscented body moisturizer.

To Wig or Not to Wig?

It's a personal question. They were too hot and itchy for me, and I was nervous they would fly off if I shook my head too hard, but I know so many women who love wigs. There are two types of wigs: real hair and synthetic. The cost is higher than you would imagine. Wigs made from real hair are the most expensive; synthetic wigs are less expensive and easier to care for, according to a wig-salon owner I spoke with. Many patients make it an outing, taking a friend along and sitting in a wig salon trying on wig after wig. One survivor friend said she became a different person when she went out with a certain wig on. It became almost like a game. For some, their hair is so important that they can't bear to let that go. If that is you, make an appointment at a wig salon at least a couple of weeks before treatment. If you can't find a local wig salon, check the American Cancer Society's TLC (Tender Loving Care) website or request a catalog. The TLC program sells wigs, along with wig accessories, scarves, turbans, and hats, and also provides free wigs to patients in need. The Pantene Beautiful Lengths program (and other programs, too) uses real, donated hair to make wigs for cancer patients (see Resources for contact information).

If finances are the only thing holding you back from a wig, there are plenty of nonprofits that can help fund a wig. Some health insurance companies will cover the cost if a doctor prescribes it as a "cranial prosthesis." Medicare and Medicaid have their own policies, so be sure to ask. (See Resources for more information.)

Another option is a wig that uses your own hair, called a

Hair Diva Halo Wig. The website gives detailed instructions about how to cut and send your own hair before you lose any of it to chemo, and the company sews your hair to a cloth cap to create a custom wig. (If you have short hair, they will supplement hair you send, but you can also have a friend or family member donate their hair.) The wig has to be worn under a hat or scarf, but if you love your real hair it might be worth the investment. (See Resources for more information.)

If hair loss is making you anxious, it's worth asking your oncologist about prevention. The latest science in preventing hair loss during chemotherapy has led to the use of something called a "cold cap." The patient wears a tight-fitting cap that is cold (15 to 40 degrees below zero Fahrenheit) before, during, and after chemotherapy treatment. The cold temperatures narrow the blood vessels underneath the scalp, which reduces the amount of chemotherapy drugs that end up in the hair follicles. With less damage to the hair follicles, theoretically less hair will fall out. I know two women who used them, and they kept most of their hair; it was patchy in spots, but it didn't fall out completely. Although used in Europe since the 1970s, cold caps were still in the trial stage in the United States until recently. In December 2015, the DigniCap Scalp Cooling System was approved by the FDA for use in adult cancer patients. The caps may or may not be covered by insurance; the estimated cost for use during treatment is $1,500 to $3,000 per patient, according to the manufacturer, Dignitana. (See Resources.)

Cold caps are not universally recommended, however. Many oncologists worry that the caps prevent the chemotherapy drugs from reaching the scalp area, which could leave some cancer cells behind. It's another item to discuss with your oncology team.

Get Back to Your Roots: Dyeing Your Hair

I am a fake blonde and have been for years. So when my hair grew back, it also turned into my original mousy brunette (with a lot of gray!). I was desperate to look like my old self (as my kids kept reminding me), so I talked to my radiation oncologist about hair dye. She recommended waiting at least six months after the end of treatment before dyeing my hair (or getting perms or using any straightening techniques).

And even after those six months, my hair stylist recommended only organic hair color. I deviated from this once, and my scalp burned from the hair dye, so just be selective about what you use; don't dump bleach on your delicate scalp! (You might try a patch test: put a little hair dye on your arm first to see if you have any sort of reaction.) Be gentle with your hair as it grows back: Skip hair dryers, curling irons, and hair rollers, and use a soft-bristle brush as your hair grows back in. It might be thicker, curlier, straighter, or the same. Everyone is different.

PLANNING FOR PARENTHOOD: FERTILITY PRESERVATION

For women, many cancer treatments can cause infertility and premature menopause, and certain cancers can make pregnancy difficult or impossible. For men, chemotherapy, radiation, and certain surgeries can affect sperm count, testosterone production, and ultimately fertility. If you're a cancer patient and you hope to have children at some point—or additional children—it's imperative to consider your fertility preservation options (150,000 Americans under forty-five are diagnosed with cancer each year, according to the American Cancer Society). Your age and the type of cancer and treatment you get all determine the fertility risks.

Any fertility conversation needs to happen early—the good news is that fertility counseling is more common than ever before. Even if you're young (reproductively speaking), you still might face fertility issues, so it's better to discuss them now rather than put it off to a time when you may be facing bigger challenges. It's essential to discuss your options with a doctor who is familiar with the subject. Some larger medical centers have entire teams devoted to what is called reproductive endocrinology and infertility, or you can find individual specialists like endocrinologists and urologists who may be able to help. There's also a developing field called oncofertility—a term created by the Feinberg School of Medicine at Northwestern University—that helps patients explore and plan for their fertility options before, during, and after cancer treatment. Also keep in mind that if you are diagnosed and have to begin treatment immediately, you might still have fertility preservation options—some fertility clinics offer what they call "rapid response," so don't panic.

For women, there are three common fertility preservation options, which involve their eggs, embryos, or ovarian tissue. Freezing eggs is the most common procedure, but it can be expensive. The process begins with fertility drugs and then random-start ovarian stimulation, which involves stimulating a woman's egg production and preserving the eggs (through a process called cryopreservation) in ten to fourteen days. This costs about $13,000 plus yearly storage fees. (Cancer treatment must usually be postponed until after the eggs are harvested.) Embyros can also be frozen; it involves ovarian stimulation followed by in vitro fertilization (IVF) using sperm from a partner or donor. This costs about $13,000 plus yearly storage fees. Freezing, and transplanting, ovarian tissue is a newer, experimental option that does not require a significant delay in cancer treatment. It involves removing one ovary then freezing the ovarian tissue until the woman has finished her cancer treatment and is ready to get pregnant. At that point, the tissue is transplanted back into her body. This method costs about $10,000 plus storage fees. Before committing to one method, do your homework; each one has pros and cons as well as varying efficacy rates.

For men, freezing sperm (called sperm banking) is the most common fertility option and is available for any male who has gone through puberty; it costs about $1,000. Another option for men undergoing radiation treatment is the use of a radiation shield to protect the testicles and help preserve sperm production. Two experimental options are testicular sperm extraction and testicular tissue freezing. There are many foundations and nonprofits that specialize in these areas, and some that can help with support, both emotional and financial (see Resources for a complete list).

Be aware that infertility might require further steps that are available through assisted reproductive technology.

ART encompasses methods of getting pregnant through artificial or partially artificial means, including embryo or egg donors, IVF, and even use of a surrogate. These methods are expensive—IVF, for example, costs between $12,000 and $20,000 per cycle. When you're already facing the cost of cancer treatment, that can be overwhelming. Some states require insurance companies to cover some costs of reproductive assistance for people facing infertility, so check with your health insurance company. If the services aren't covered, you can still submit the claim and prepare to appeal if it's denied. Patient navigators can be very helpful with this process; be sure to ask your hospital or medical center to connect you with one if you're facing this sort of complex insurance situation. In addition, some fertility centers and individual doctors will give discounts to cancer patients, so if you're researching fertility centers ask about any pricing options available.

Adoption or fostering might be another option for you and your family, and both are worth exploring.

If you have been diagnosed with cancer while you are pregnant, seek out a specialist. This topic needs a whole book on its own, but an excellent resource to start with is Hope for Two, a website devoted exclusively to pregnant women with cancer (see Resources).

Cancer by the Numbers

Three years after my diagnosis, I made a list of what I had been through. Sometimes numbers speak louder than words.

- 4 hospitalizations
- 5 mammograms
- 7 ultrasounds
- 12 CT scans
- 2 PET scans
- 4 PET/CT combo scans
- 4 bone scans
- 40 days of radiation therapy
- 15 chemotherapy infusions
- 500-ish days of the PARP-inhibitor oral chemo clinical trial drug veliparib (ABT-888)
- Unknown hours of sitting in plastic waiting room chairs
- Unknown hours sitting in exam rooms in pink paper gowns (open to the front)
- 300-ish forms filled out
- 2 general practitioners visited
- 5 oncologists consulted
- 2 radiation oncologists
- 3 surgeries
- 2 breasts removed

- 19 lymph nodes removed
- 90-ish sutures
- 2 saline breast implants inserted
- 2 breast surgeons
- 2 plastic surgeons
- 1 gynecological oncology surgeon
- 1 gynecological surgeon resident
- 2 anesthesiologists
- 1 dermatologist
- 1 oncology psychiatrist
- 1 psychologist
- 1 physical therapist
- 1 oncology social worker
- 3 therapeutic massage therapists
- Untold number of amazing nurses
- 1 mean nurse
- 1 completely inept nurse
- 1 fine needle aspiration (FNA)
- 1 rib biopsy
- 1 PICC line inserted into my arm
- 1 PICC line removal
- 1 chest port insertion
- 1 chest port removal

- 500-ish blood draws
- 50-plus IV lines in my arms
- 2 IV lines in my foot
- 1 IV line in my neck
- 1 catheter
- 5 medical centers visited
- Many, many milligrams of many, many antibiotics, narcotics, painkillers, and other assorted pills and creams
- 2 clinical drug trials
- 1 clinical drug trial canceled
- 1 individual clinical drug trial
- 10-plus days of fasting
- 6 marijuana cookies consumed
- 2 hospital beds set up in my bedroom
- Countless liters of potassium fluid administered
- Unknown number of wheelchair rides
- 600-plus prescriptions filled
- 1 hospital meal actually consumed
- 50 airline flights
- Unknown number of bags of pretzels eaten
- A handful of amazing flight attendants
- 1 mean flight attendant (yes, I'm talking to you, Jennifer, at a major airline)

- Many glasses of wine and champagne (depending on the month and trial status)

- 100-plus pizzas consumed

- 3 head shavings

- 12 silk scarves

- 1 itchy wig

- 4 visits to church

- 2,000 prayers

- 1,000 readings of the flower pot in my bedroom that says HOPE

- Unknown hours of bad television

- 300-plus homemade meals dropped at our doorstep

- 300-plus cards of encouragement

- Countless voice mail messages with words of encouragement

- Countless conversations and emails and hugs with the bravest cancer patients and survivors imaginable

- 1 incredibly diligent husband and family who wouldn't take no for an answer

- 2 children who took my breath away every minute (plus 3 amazing, loving nieces)

- Buckets of tears

- Hundreds of laughs

- Endless kindness

That was my list. Make your own here:

_____

_____

_____

_____

_____

_____

_____

_____

_____

_____

_____

_____

_____

_____

_____

_____

_____

_____

_____

_____

CHAPTER 7

HORIZONTAL, OR: HOW TO SLEEP

Western culture seems to view sleep as a luxury, equating "sleeping in" or taking naps with laziness. This is scientifically misguided, particularly when you're talking about someone who's sick. We all need sleep to recover every night, and it's even more important when you are ill. Your body heals during sleep—it's that simple. A few things that happen while you sleep: Your heart and blood vessels repair and heal; your brain forms, fixes, and maintains new pathways (neurons); and your immune system gets ready to fight infection. Naps are crucial, too. And, again, fatigue—the kind of tired that isn't fixed with sleep—is often a side effect of cancer treatment. Side effects of lack of sleep (increased blood pressure, lower insulin resistance, weakened immune system, as well as intensification of some other conditions like depression and memory loss) can make your road trip even more complicated.

INSOMNIA (I'M WIDE AWAKE)

Insomnia comes with the territory in Cancerland. Combine a set of drugs, an anxiety-producing diagnosis, possibly physical pain, and you're set up for some sleep-deprived nights. (I was up at 4:00 AM on some nights, puttering around or writing or folding laundry, then going back to bed at 6:00 AM and sleeping until noon. You just have to go with it.) Cancer patients often have a reverse sleep schedule: You sleep during the day and are awake at night. Do what you can to normalize your schedule with the goal of maximizing sleep. But don't discount lack of sleep; if you suffer from insomnia it's incredibly important to mention it to your doctor so you can find a way to get proper rest.

FATIGUE

Exhaustion is a common side effect of cancer treatment; it's hard to avoid no matter what type of cancer you have. The medications and the sheer mental weight of a cancer diagnosis can slow you down physically; doctors generally measure your white blood cell count (noted as WBC on your chart) to evaluate your fatigue. White blood cells fight infection in the body—a healthy body produces about one hundred billion new cells every day—and chemotherapy and radiation destroy these cells. (These particular white blood cells are called neutrophils, and neutropenia is what results when too few of them exist in the body.) Extremely low WBC levels can also lead to frequent bruising and anemia. Fatigue can cause you to feel slightly sleepy or like you cannot get out of bed; it varied for me, but all I knew was I needed a nap every single afternoon. What is most frustrating about fatigue is its invisibility: Talking about it doesn't necessarily mean anyone takes it seriously.

A few things were recommended to me to help ease the fatigue, including exercise and certain foods. Nothing worked for me while I was in treatment. I tried to walk every day—even just around the block—when I felt up to it, but some days I was just wiped out and could only manage a walk around the house. There are many exceptions, obviously; some people bike, jog, and feel up to active workouts while in treatment. But as long as you keep moving in some capacity, you shouldn't feel pressure to take a jog or a five-mile bike ride. I had practiced yoga for over ten years, and during that time I couldn't even fathom getting into the downward-dog pose. It's important to listen to your body on those days and not push it; your body is working overtime to try and metabolize the treatment, and forcing it to work even harder isn't the best solution. Making time in your day to rest is really the only remedy, and accepting that you're slowing down (if only temporarily) is part of the treatment.

However, that isn't a prescription to spend the entire day in bed or on the couch. Mobility is important, even if it's just walking around the house to build up strength until you can then stroll to the mailbox, and then maybe even down the street (with supervision!). Just be kind to yourself. Discuss severe mobility issues with your doctor; there might be alternative ways for you to exercise. (For more on exercise both during and after treatment, see Move It in chapter 10 and Recurrence in chapter 12.)

COUNTING SHEEP AND OTHER SLEEP AIDS

If you have persistent sleep issues, talk to your doctor about medications that might be helpful in the short-term. Don't take anything—whether over-the-counter (Typlenol PM), herbal (melatonin), or prescription (Ambien, Belsomra, or Lunesta)—without talking to your oncologist. You don't want any medication mishaps.

To increase the odds of a good night's sleep, try these bedtime rituals:

- Don't type, text, watch TV, or use your laptop or electronic device within one hour of bedtime. The screen triggers brain activity, or cognitive stimulation, which is the exact opposite of what you want when you're trying to sleep.

- Make sure the temperature in your bedroom is comfortable. The ideal sleeping temperature is 65 degrees Fahrenheit. It's better to have it slightly cold than too warm.

- Don't listen to loud music right before bed.

- Don't drink caffeine or alcohol within a few hours of bedtime; they can both act as stimulants.

- Get up at the same time every morning even if you didn't sleep through the night.

- Try a sound machine. White noise, birdsong, or ocean sounds can be peaceful and soothe you into sleep.

- If your room lets in a lot of natural light, try new shades or blinds, or a nice soft sleep mask for your eyes. (Cotton is best if you're having night sweats; it's easy on your skin and you can throw it in the wash.)

- Meditate before bedtime. I used to joke that it felt like cheating to meditate while on the amount of prescription medications I was taking. But if you like to meditate and feel up to it, try it in a dark, quiet room before falling asleep.

- If you go to bed and can't fall asleep after twenty minutes, get up, do something for a few minutes in another room, then come back and try again.

CHAPTER 8

THERE IS NO PRIZE FOR THE BEST PATIENT

Taking care of yourself as a patient requires two things: asking for help, and taking the time to do things for you. Forget the medical side; the cancer road trip requires so much more than just medicine. Medicine is just the gas in the tank. But what person in their right mind starts a road trip without a bag of snacks, drinks, maps, electronic devices, headphones, and a few Band-Aids? Only a moron.

At every appointment, your doctor will use your vital signs as a benchmark to influence everything that comes after—for example, if your blood pressure rises or your weight drops significantly, your treatment won't progress as business-as-usual. The basic tests described in the next section are not only physical signs of life but emotional signs as well—the ways of making the road trip palatable, which is vital to life as a patient. Vital, as in essential. Whatever you need to make your day, your week, your month more tolerable, you should ask for it. You will suffer enough both physically and emotionally that it'll be imperative that you ask for whatever will make you feel good—the meaning of "within reason" can shift dramatically when you have cancer. A drive to your favorite beach or mountain, a visit to the driving range, a stack of travel magazines, a trip to the mall—everyone has different soul-soothing techniques. This isn't the time to be bashful about it.

VITAL SIGNS: HOW TO ASK FOR HELP

Since there is no pot of gold waiting for the most cooperative and quiet patient, ask for what you need. If the doctor has her hand on the door handle, ready to move on to the next patient, don't be afraid to stop her and ask a burning question. I was known to open the exam room door, half-naked in my paper gown, and call out to a doctor walking down the hall or ask a passing nurse when the team was going to see me. My sister and my husband also wrote emails to various doctors at all hours. Make yourself heard. Ask politely and respectfully, but firmly. Medical professionals are typically terrific, but they often won't do anything outside their scheduled agendas unless you ask. Be the squeaky wheel.

Here are some other tips to make life as a patient a tiny bit easier:

- Make a list of questions before each doctor's appointment, and be ready to go through all of them. Don't feel rushed by their time schedule. Ask your caregivers for input, too; they often see things you don't.

- Make a spreadsheet or chart to keep track of your medications. Not because you don't trust your family and closest friends to track the myriad drugs that you will take, but . . . really, you shouldn't trust them, or yourself, to remember the milligrams and dosage and drug names with six syllables and too many consonants. Include the dosage and drug name on the spreadsheet, as well as any special instructions such as "take with food." For post-operative drugs, you must record the time you took the pill and the dosage. This is usually on a twenty-four-hour clock—or military time—which can be confusing. If you're unsure, have a caregiver or friend help you. You cannot mess around with the timing of a dosage. Print out the chart and hang it on the refrigerator, keeping one copy by your bedside and one in your appointment bag. (See page 266 for a sample medication chart.)

- Find a twenty-four-hour pharmacy (with a drive-through window, if possible), even if it's a few miles out of your way. You never know when you'll need a medication or need a friend to pick something up for you. (Silver lining: The 1:00 AM pharmacy visit is always good for people-watching.)

- Rotate your spots. You will be spending a lot of time in your house or apartment, so don't spend all your time in one place. Boredom and frustration are increased by looking at the same old view all day and all night; try to take a day on the sofa, a day in your bed, a day in the chair by the window. Fresh air is also important! Make sure you can open a window and let the air in, even if it's just a crack.

Have a friend or family member start researching resources that might be useful. Make a long list and include everything you think you might need to get you through treatment and into recovery, even if you end up crossing most of it off. In the beginning you have no idea how this road trip is going to go, and the medical world focuses on medical things, so you have to dig up these kinds of resources yourself. Consider services such as local meal delivery—they can be a godsend (or even a lifeline), and many meal delivery companies can ship meals to your doorstep. If you're traveling for treatment, there are nonprofits that coordinate free flights on private jets for patients and their families (Corporate Angel Network, for example; see Resources for more information). There are even cancer couples' retreats run by nonprofits that you and your partner can take (see Resources). All of these things are out there and can help make the cancer experience just a little bit easier, but you have to find them and use them. (I've included as many as I could in the Resources section, but there are many more to uncover.)

SLAP ON A LITTLE LIPSTICK: SMALL PICK-ME-UPS

This is the time to enjoy the little things. Getting your makeup done to hide any dark circles or fill in missing eyebrows, trying a new lipstick or a new shirt, buying a new album that you rock out to. These are not luxuries—they are essentials to keep your head up and your thoughts on getting through it.

- MINI-MAKEOVERS: Many makeup counters and beauty stores offer free mini-makeover sessions. If you need something to perk you up, pop in for a fifteen-minute makeover. I always explained to the makeup artist that I was in treatment so she would use gentler products; I found people were so kind and really wanted to help. There are also many national programs that participate in "makeover days" or have programs for cancer patients. Seeing yourself in the mirror during treatment can be unsettling; but somehow with a little mascara and lipstick, and a little kindness, the day can seem a tiny bit better. The power of makeup can be surprising: Claudia Poccia, the president and CEO of Gurwitch Products, which owns the Laura Mercier brand of beauty products, watched her sister struggle with her appearance during her battle with ovarian cancer. Poccia gave her a Laura Mercier "Bonne Mine" makeup kit, and she wore the makeup every day. This prompted Poccia and co-founder Laura Mercier to set up a fund for research and education for ovarian cancer (see Resources for more info), and profits from the sale of certain Laura Mercier products go to the fund.

- FACIALS: If you feel up to it and your doctor hasn't advised you otherwise, get a facial. I have an aesthetician friend, and she would just gently rub my face with organic herbs and creams; it was more about being comforted and pampered than getting my face clean. (Just be sure they don't use any chemical peels, lasers, or similar procedures that might interfere with treatment.)

- MANICURES AND PEDICURES: If you're determined to keep your toes and nails looking good through treatment, invest in your own set of nail tools to bring to the nail salon and make sure to thoroughly clean them afterward. (Skip acrylic nail fillers, however; they are not advised during treatment.) Chemotherapy can affect your fingernails, toenails, and nail beds—the color and sensitivity can change, so make sure you're being gentle on your hands. Wear rubber gloves if you're washing any dishes (you shouldn't be!) to prevent nail fungal infections. (See Chemo Side Effects in chapter 4 for more information.)

Quotes That Won't Irritate You

People will send you a lot of "inspirational" books and quotes when they find out you're sick. The following were the least annoying to me (and actually cheered me up a bit).

Never, never, never give up.
—Winston Churchill

What counts is not necessarily the size of the dog in the fight—
it's the size of the fight in the dog.
—President Dwight D. Eisenhower

While there's life there is hope.
—Stephen Hawking

Apparently, there is nothing that cannot happen today.
—Mark Twain

Once you choose hope, anything is possible.
—Christopher Reeve

God turns you from one feeling to another and teaches you
by means of opposites, so that you will have two wings to fly,
not one.
—Rumi

There is always a before and an after.
My advice, travel light. Choose only what you need most to see
you through.
—Alice Hoffman, *Survival Lessons*

Attitude is a little thing that makes a big difference.
—Winston Churchill

There are only two ways to live your life.
One is as though nothing is a miracle.
The other is as though everything is a miracle.
—Albert Einstein

Some days there won't be a song in your heart. Sing anyway.
—Emory Austin

If you are going through hell, keep going.
—Winston Churchill

One life on this Earth is all we get, whether it is enough or not
enough, and the obvious conclusion would seem to be that at
the very least we are fools if we do not live it as fully and bravely
and beautifully as we can.
—Frederick Buechner

It is not really necessary to look too far into the future; we see
enough already to be certain it will be magnificent. Only let us
hurry and open the roads.
—Wilbur Wright

To say yes to life is at one and the same time to say yes
to oneself.
—Dag Hammarskjöld

The world breaks everyone, and afterward many are strong
at the broken places.
—Ernest Hemingway

CHAPTER 9

THE FAMILY

PARENTING WITH CANCER, OR PACKING LUNCHES WHILE BALD

It's one thing to be a patient and quite another to be a patient and a mom. Remember that old cliché, "Moms don't get sick days"? Surprise! They do, and the whole family changes because of it. Adjusting to a new role—even if it's temporary—is frustrating and fraught with complications. Add your illness, plus your spouse's emotions, plus the kids, and it's one giant, unsolvable math equation. I was completely unprepared for the ways cancer would change my life as a parent. Lying in bed (our bedroom was down a few stairs, under the kitchen), unable to move, listening to the world upstairs—I could hear the kitchen faucet turning on and off, the opening and closing of the cupboards as oatmeal was being made and snacks and lunches packed. I felt utterly helpless. And people would say, "It's your job to just get better," but it doesn't feel like a job—it feels exhausting and leechlike and frustrating and dismal. So I would listen to the life going on upstairs and cry.

Tragically, parenting with a cancer diagnosis is not uncommon. Almost 3 million children in the United States have, or have had, a parent diagnosed with cancer, according to the American Academy of Child and Adolescent Psychiatry (AACAP). The American Cancer Society estimates that more than 367,000 parents with children under the age of eighteen were diagnosed with invasive cancer in 2014. Put another way, 1 in 5 adults diagnosed with cancer in 2013 have children under the age of 18, according to the AACAP. That translates to a lot of families faced with the task of keeping the household functioning while going through what is often one of the scariest experiences of their lives.

What struck me was that the tiniest parenting details— taking the kids to get their hair cut, organizing a birthday party, or signing up for ballet class—ended up being the ones that made me feel the most disconnected. (And those were the details that I was afraid would be forgotten by everyone should I not make it.) Being healthy enough to take care of those things made me feel like I was back in the world: the homework packet, the karate class, the cookies for the class holiday party. Those are the details that make up so much of childhood. When I felt crappy, I got creative: I watched cooking shows with my daughter when I was too sick to read to her, discussing which dish we should try or which contestant was the best; or I listened to the kids talk about their day while I brushed their hair. Those seemingly insignificant things, the smallest moments, will create micro-memories for you and the kids to think about during the bad days.

Besides the fear of leaving my kids (i.e., dying), the hardest thing for me as a mom with cancer was being told to stay away from my sick children while I was in treatment. Just when you want to hold them and comfort them, sick kids are exposing you to infection. It will break your heart, but you must stay away. Be sure to tell the school and teacher what is going on so they can warn you about any nasty illnesses going around. The last thing you need is a case of pinkeye or bronchitis in the middle of treatment.

You also cannot take the kids to the pediatrician, even if it's a healthy-child checkup; the risk of infection is too high. Arrange for your spouse or partner or a grandparent to take them to any appointments. Make sure you tell your pediatrician about your situation; it's important for them to know for the child's medical record (particularly if your cancer involves a genetic element). It's also essential for them to know in terms of vaccines; patients undergoing chemotherapy cannot be exposed to live viruses, for example, which can affect vaccination schedules. Also, if the flu shot is not widely available due to a shortage, certain doses may be available to you (and your family) since you are immunocompromised. After the kids come back from a doctor's visit, make sure they wash their hands thoroughly and change their clothes, placing the dirty clothes in the washing machine. This can reduce the risk of any germs carried into the house.

Last practical tip for parenting in treatment: make sure you have help changing diapers! Changing a diaper while having chemo-induced nausea is not recommended. If you want to participate (or there is a diaper emergency), be sure to wear disposable rubber gloves to protect against germs.

The physicality of parenting is often overlooked, especially with little kids. Physically being with your kids can be a challenge for a parent with cancer, whether you're recovering at home from chemo, radiation, or surgery, or your treatment involves long hospital stays. (Talk to your doctors about having your kids visit if you'll be in the hospital for more than a week.) Talking to your kids about what you can do, rather than what you can't do, is one strategy. Things like: Daddy can't lift you up in the air, but he can still tickle you; or, Mommy can't walk you to school, but she can still read to you.

I was very concerned about not hugging and holding my kids after my double mastectomy/salpingo-oophorectomy and reconstruction (and even after more basic procedures like the portacath insertion). It was impossible for the kids to get in bed with me without pulling something out or knocking something over! But a generous employee at the University of California San Francisco Cancer Care Center shared a tip I will always treasure: The kids might be nervous, especially about seeing you in pain, so to encourage physical contact place six or seven pillows on a comfortable floor and sit in the middle. (Hold pillows near your surgical sites, too.) Then ask, encourage, or cajole the kids to come sit with you and snuggle; your body will be protected if they shift or move too quickly, and they get to be with you (and you get to smell their lovely heads and feel their warm bodies).

Eventually you get into a family groove—that dreaded phrase, "the new normal"—and things seem more manageable, at least more than they are in the beginning when the wheels are coming off the bus.

Here are my top cancer mom insights:

- You will cry the first time your child reaches for the babysitter instead of you.

- "Fake it till you make it" is what sustains you as a cancer parent. It works 90 percent of the time, like when you're dragging yourself to the dinner table or watching the kids in the bath. But don't beat yourself up about the other 10 percent.

- Have a strategy. If I could sit with the kids from 4:00 PM to 7:00 PM I counted it as a victory. (That shifted depending on when my treatment was, like when I switched to mornings.) Some weeks I was too sick in the mornings and exhausted later in the night; you have to roll with it. A survivor friend told me she did mornings; her goal was to get up with the kids, make breakfast, pack lunches, and get them to school. And then she had backup for the afternoons and evenings. Just pick something that works for you and the family—a schedule will give everyone some structure in what can be anything but certain times.

- You will become acutely aware of how many moms die in movies and television shows. Try to pre-screen the choices so you're not caught silently crying while watching something with the kids.

- You will miss certain events with your kids while you're in treatment. It's just a fact. You cannot take them to birth-day parties (or throw them one) if you're in chemo; the risk of getting sick while your immune system is compro-mised is too high. You cannot go anywhere large groups of kids gather; no playgrounds, no trampoline parks, no arcades, no mini-golf. But tell yourself you will be there for other things and other moments.

- Listening to someone else parent your child—whether it's a spouse, family member, or other caregiver—can be excruciating. So many survivor moms I spoke to said the same thing: You have to let it go. You can make lists and verbalize how you do (or did) things (such as, Charlie only eats spaghetti with butter, but Janna likes spaghetti with tomato sauce). But once someone else is on duty, you have to close your eyes and trust that they will be as good you are. You have to conserve your energy, and worrying about whether your spouse will make sure the kids have packed a water bottle isn't the best use of your energy when you're recovering from the latest chemo cycle or tending to radiation burns.

- Take advantage of the good days. Don't waste your energy on cleaning out the refrigerator; use it to do something special with the kids. When I had a burst of energy or had a "day off" from feeling terrible, I took my kids to their favorite spots: the ice cream shop, a ferry boat ride, or to a movie. It was my special time with them, time to reconnect and check in. Even if it was just an hour or two,

I wanted to create good memories that might cancel out the memories of me lying in bed for so many months.

- Consider taking your child to a therapist (particularly if they are suddenly acting out or exhibiting any unusual behavior like pulling out their hair or showing appetite or sleep changes). They are going through a trauma, too, and there is a lot of turmoil and a lot to discuss surrounding the word *cancer*. In my case, I had no idea how to even approach the topic with my then five-year-old daughter, and I was terrified of saying the wrong thing. We got a referral and took her to see a local child psychiatrist, and it helped us all so much to have someone outside the immediate circle navigating the conversation with us. The ages of the kids matter: Different ages have different emotional needs, of course, so keep that in mind when finding a therapist. A teenager will be seeking comfort and answers on a far different level than a seven-year-old will. Individual therapy (rather than support groups)—whether it's with a clinical social worker, psychologist, or child psychiatrist—is usually recommended for kids.

- Try to keep things as routine as possible for the kids. Routine is a comfort, particularly for small children.

- Obviously a recurrence of cancer is everyone's worst fear, and for a child it can be overwhelming. Be sure to seek out support for your kids if that happens, so you can have a few phrases to use when the kids start asking big questions (or even hinting at them).

Talking to Kids about Cancer

This was one of the hardest moments in the entire cancer experience: What were we going to say to our daughter, who was only five at the time? (Our son was too young to understand.) I was absolutely paralyzed at the thought and terrified of saying the wrong thing. Here are a few basics I learned from books, therapists, and a child psychiatrist we met with. While you may have to adjust the language based on your children's ages, the basics remain the same. And prepare yourself: As insane as it sounds, you need to keep it together for the conversation. A parent in tears is not the most comforting sight to a child.

- Don't make any promises, particularly when you've just been diagnosed. Promising them that Mommy or Daddy won't die, or won't be sick forever, does not help them; it will only confuse them and make them more upset if the situation changes.

- Make sure your family and friends are all on the same page about what is being communicated to the kids. Send out an email if you need to, giving the parameters of what you have told them. The last thing you need is a family friend or Aunt Betty telling your son that "Mommy/Daddy is really, really sick," or something equally as upsetting.

- Try to communicate exactly what is going on. Telling your kids that on this day you get this medicine and then you go the hospital on this day helps give them a framework. And preparing them for any physical changes can be helpful.

- Little kids have big ears. As in, watch what you say when you think they aren't listening.

- Tell them that you have cancer. Use the actual word. Don't say, "sick," "boo-boo," or "under the weather." Kids are literal, and they need to know that what you have is not the same as their stomach flu. (And they won't understand why you aren't getting better as quickly as they do when they cut their finger.)

- Make sure to mention the fact that they can't "catch" cancer, that it is not contagious.

- Acknowledge their emotions and encourage them to share them. Some kids get angry; you can help guide their anger by saying something like, "I'm mad, too! I'm so mad I got cancer and it keeps me from being at your soccer practice/ dance class/piano recital." Or, "I know you're mad that we had to cancel our trip to the beach. I'm so glad you told me that. But as soon as I feel better we will make another plan."

- Expect their emotions to change. Your kids might react one way during one phase of your treatment then react differently when you enter another phase. Just be ready.

- Tell them it's not their fault. Some kids, particularly younger kids, might think they did something to cause your illness or make you go away from them (if you have to spend chunks of time in the hospital or travel for treatment). Make it very clear that nothing they did caused you to get cancer.

- Be ready for their questions. Kids come up with things you can't even imagine. I'll never forget the day my daughter asked me, "When are your boobies going to grow back?" I think I literally pulled the car over I was so shocked! But remember, it's better that they are engaged and curious and feel comfortable asking you questions than completely shutting down.

Kids' Books That Help Explain, "Mommy or Daddy Has Cancer"

Butterfly Kisses and Wishes on Wings—When Someone You Love Has Cancer . . . a Hopeful, Helpful Book for Kids by **Ellen McVicker:**
This beautifully illustrated, award-winning book is told through the voice of a child and shows how children can be with their mom who is going through cancer (the type of cancer is unspecified). Also available in Spanish.

Let My Colors Out by **Courtney Filigenzi:**
A young boy deals with his mother's illness by using colors for his emotions. A good picture book for young kids with a parent who is in treatment, and one of the few books that features a boy as the main character.

Mom and the Polka-Dot Boo-Boo by **Eileen Sutherland:**
Written by a breast cancer survivor and mother, the story explains breast cancer to young children. Illustrated by Sutherland's daughter.

Mom Has Cancer! by **Jennifer Moore-Mallinos:**
Aimed at preschoolers and young children, this picture book

encourages kids to express their feelings about a mom who is undergoing treatment.

My Parent Has Cancer and It Really Sucks by Maya Silver and Marc Silver:

Written by the daughter and husband of a breast cancer patient, this is the first book specifically aimed at teenagers who are living with a parent undergoing treatment. A blend of advice from kids and medical professionals and a section for parents to help guide discussions with their teenager.

Nowhere Hair by Sue Glader:

This picture book follows a little girl who knows her mom's hair is gone but tries to find out why. A modern take on explaining cancer to kids under eight.

Our Mom Has Cancer by Abigail Ackermann and Adrienne Ackermann:

Two siblings wrote about the year their mother went through breast cancer treatment. Appropriate for preschoolers through third graders.

Our Mom Is Getting Better and *Our Dad Is Getting Better* by Alex Silver, Emily Silver, and Anna Rose Silver:

These two titles were written by three children (and siblings) who explain their mother's treatment and recovery from breast cancer as well as a father's cancer treatment and recovery. Both books are for children ages four to nine whose parents have survived cancer treatment.

What's Up with Bridget's Mom? Medikidz Explain Breast Cancer by Kim Chilman-Blair:

A graphic novel aimed at kids twelve and over, this book uses a group of superheroes to explain breast cancer. Part of the

"Medikidz" series, other topics available include explaining leukemia, brain tumors, colorectal cancer, osteosarcoma, melanoma,
prostate cancer, and lung cancer. Also available in Spanish.

When Someone You Know Has Cancer:
An Activity Booklet for Families:

PBS Kids, WGBH, children's book author and illustrator Marc
Brown, and the Livestrong Foundation joined together to create
this online booklet that helps kids talk about cancer in the family.
Using Brown's popular book and television character Arthur, the
booklet addresses cancer in parents and grandparents for kids
ages three to ten. You can print the booklet directly from the web
link; also available in Spanish.

http://www-tc.pbskids.org/arthur/health/pdf/arthur_cancer_
english.pdf

You Are the Best Medicine by Julie Aigner Clark:

A picture book for ages two to six, written by a cancer survivor,
that shows how kids can still be themselves around a sick parent.
The patient is a mother and the main character is her daughter;
the type of cancer is not specified. Be prepared to cry.

"YOU TAKE OUT THE GARBAGE," OR: CANCER AND MARRIAGE

People say that cancer changes everything. But the biggest
surprise to me was how little it changed things with my husband. There is a period of crisis, of course, when you're clutch-
ing each other's hands and can't bear to think of the "till
death do us part" vow actually coming true. It seems almost
unspeakable. But then, possibly out of necessity, you just keep
on with the familiar: Tuesdays are garbage night, a leaky faucet needs fixing, eye exams and dental appointments need to

be made. My husband and I squeezed out a few date nights to the movies or to dinner, which helped us pretend for a little while that nothing was changing. The marriage marches on, from the mundane to the magical and back again.

Hopefully your partner will be there to hold your hand during appointments, or make you laugh when the time is right, or sit quietly when you just want someone to sit with. But they might not, and that's normal. They might want to take a walk or a bike ride or just drive around and have some time to themselves. What few people talk about is this: Even with cancer you will still nag your spouse about taking out the garbage. There will still be moments—weeks, months even—of an ordinary marriage. Cancer doesn't mean a rosy glow on everything, sweet smiles at every turn. A cancer diagnosis merely adds another element to the otherwise complicated act of marriage.

Making sure your partner or spouse gets time off is important. Their life has been turned upside down, as well. And they might be the one with the health insurance, so they simply must go to work every day to keep the insurance and the income. If you, the patient, are the breadwinner, that pressure will undoubtedly be even worse. (And that might require a financial planning meeting; see Resources for financial planning options.) I can say from the other side that it's best to get your feelings out; this isn't the time to let resentment build. Talking to a therapist or marriage counselor, even if it's once or twice, can be a lifesaver. If your spouse or partner's family is able to visit, that can provide some relief and comfort for them. Your partner's in Cancerland, too, albeit on a different level; they need someone to turn to as well. Allowing them to lose it and cry—in front of you or alone or with whomever they trust—is so important. They need that space, particularly if you're facing a prolonged treatment. (One caveat here: If your in-laws create more stress for you, the patient, plan accordingly so your partner can have time alone with their family.)

What I felt most those first three months of my cancer road trip was anger. This was totally unexpected. It stemmed from so many places: anger that there might be a life without me being present, anger that my husband didn't understand my emotions and exactly what I was going through, anger at this life interruption that might possibly be longer than a pause. Knowing ahead of time that there might be a level of anger would have helped me. Being able to tell your partner that it's cancer you're angry with, rather than them or the over-scrambled eggs they made you, is imperative.

Your partner or spouse also might not want to talk about your diagnosis and everything that goes along with it. There might be more silence than you would like. Not everyone is ready to talk about the same things right at the same moment. It was too hard for me in the beginning to talk to my husband about my concerns, so I wrote him a letter instead. Do whatever feels right for you, but get the words out. To me it was important to get the words down, and even if we didn't have to face the unspoken right then, I knew at least I had said what I wanted to say. Ignoring the obvious and not addressing certain realities only adds to the frustration, disappointment, and anger over your illness.

Once I had finished the worst of the treatment, my husband and I went away for one night to a hotel ten minutes from our house—we were literally away for twenty-five hours. It was hard for me, emotionally, to leave the kids, but we needed the time to reconnect. The reality is that your partnership gets put on the back burner when you're in the thick of treatment, with or without kids. From the outside we looked like a regular couple, but I was different: breast expanders, no nipples, no ovaries, in menopause, exhausted—you are not the same, surgery or not, and it's important to discuss that. Added to that, I had no sex drive, so talking about anything related to sex was very uncomfortable and felt awkward, even with my husband. The time together turned out to be a wonderful escape, but it took effort and big emotional leaps I never would have anticipated.

Reduced or a complete lack of sexual intercourse is also a reality of cancer. It might last weeks, months, or even years and can greatly affect couples. Physical and emotional changes make sex a low priority, or impossible for some patients. If intercourse isn't possible, try snuggling or just hugging. Try to keep some form of intimacy going, even if it's just holding hands. I felt like less of a woman without my breasts, and I also felt a certain amount of shame in front of my husband; he had seen me in some unimaginable moments. How could he look at me in an intimate way after seeing me bloated, vomiting, and with drains sticking out of my chest? I could barely look in the mirror after my double mastectomy, much less imagine baring all in the bedroom. Male cancer patients may feel uncomfortable with missing parts or lack of sexual desire or the physical inability to have sex due to treatment. If you're diagnosed with tongue cancer, your salivary glands and your tongue itself may be affected, which makes kissing difficult. It might help to view these as setbacks, not roadblocks. The scars and feelings that left me shaking and vulnerable are now distant memories; a lot of talking and a lot of self-acceptance (and a few cute nightgowns) helped me see myself as a woman again.

And remember, your partner may feel just as nervous with you. They might not know what feels good to you, or they might be afraid to hurt you; this isn't a one-way street—it's a two-lane road, and you both have to start talking. If you can't bear to bring it up, consider talking to a sex therapist or counselor or attending a sexual health program at a hospital or medical center; having a third party might make the topic easier to discuss and address. (For more on sex after cancer, see chapter 12.)

THE BIG TALKS: WILLS AND ADVANCE MEDICAL DIRECTIVES

Part of a cancer diagnosis involves legal paperwork. As scary and surreal as it may seem, having a will in place is critical once you receive a cancer diagnosis. It doesn't make you a negative patient (or person) if you take care of these details; it makes you a smart one. A will is particularly important if you're the caregiver for someone or you are a parent or guardian of a child (or children). The guardianship of children can turn litigious, and by naming a guardian (or guardians) in a legal will, there is less chance that your wishes will be ignored by the court. (Usually when no guardian is designated by the parent or parents, the children become wards of the state. Talk to an attorney about the specific laws in your state.) Taking care of these details will let you focus on what's most important, which is treatment and doing the things you love to do. It will be hard to face these realities, especially on paper, but it's essential.

Drafting a basic will can be as simple as using an online program or asking a lawyer friend to help you. (If you have a complicated financial or family situation, get advice from a lawyer who specializes in that area.) A will must be notarized, which is a fairly easy process. If you're married, it is generally advised that you write the will with your spouse or at the very least show it to them before getting it notarized. Make sure there is a designated beneficiary. If you're in a partnership, not legally married, you need to consult a lawyer to make sure you have access to all of the legal forms.

An advance medical directive (or AMD), also known as a living will, dictates who will make medical decisions for you if you become unable, including issues such as whether you have signed a do not resuscitate (DNR) order. Although this is an optional form and not legally required before treatment, it is strongly advised that it be part of your medical record at the medical center before any procedures are done. (The definition of "procedure" varies by medical institute, so be sure to ask your doctor.) An AMD requires your signature and either a notarization or the signatures of two adult witnesses in order to be valid. Taking the time to prepare it on your terms is essential; this is not a decision you want to make with any sort of time pressure (such as the night before surgery). It is valid until you revoke it.

A health care proxy (HCP) is a type of AMD. In an HCP, you, the patient, designate one person to act as your health care "agent." (The agent must be at least eighteen years old and cannot be your physician.) The intent is to give you the authority to choose someone to speak for you when you are incapacitated. The doctors must follow the agent's wishes as if they were your own wishes.

Another small detail that can have big ramifications is writing down, or sharing, computer passwords. If your partner, spouse, or family member has a work password, they need to share that with their boss or coworkers if they'll be away from work for an extended period of time. But even passwords for the family computer or a joint bank account need to be written down or safely shared with a designated person. Particularly if you're facing a type of cancer that could affect your cognition or communication, such as brain cancer, you want to have all of these details taken care of just in case.

WE ARE FAMILY:
FAMILY DYNAMICS AND THE BIG C

Just as cancer doesn't necessarily change your marriage, it likely won't change any family dynamics, either. Finding a rhythm in the family, particularly if you have extended family or have to move in with relatives during treatment, requires some preparation. Family burnout happens. It's better to know this than to be caught off guard. I was completely oblivious about how we would handle my diagnosis and relate to each other. Relying on family as an adult comes with its own difficulties, but there are a few tips to keep in mind.

Family dynamics are based on the idea that each piece operates as part of a whole. It's not your imagination; there is a real term for it. Social scientists call it the family systems theory, where patterns develop that help the entire unit. This is helpful when you're deciding who is cooking dinner and who is in charge of the laundry, but it can also trap each family member in a role that never changes. If you are moving back home, or family is coming to live with you during treatment, remember this. You don't automatically need to revert to life as a teenager. Try shifting your approach. Treat your siblings like friends, rather than like your siblings from childhood.

Being family doesn't mean you can't have your own needs and wants, and that the "family obligation" and rules supersede everything else. You are the patient, and you need to have your voice heard. And on the flip side, even if you are the patient, you are still you. You might be a sister, brother, mother, father, aunt, uncle, or cousin. Don't let cancer rob you of your voice. It's easy to slip into what I call "patient otherness" and watch the world go on around you, without you. But you need to participate as much as you can.

CHAPTER 10

BOARDING PASS: TRAVELING WITH CANCER

For six months, I had to fly from my home in Northern California to City of Hope Medical Center in Southern California to participate in a clinical drug trial. (See Clinical Trials in chapter 4 for more information on how these work.) Whether you are forced to travel for treatment or want to plan a vacation while in treatment, this is the chapter for you.

Traveling for treatment (as opposed to taking a vacation while in treatment) brought its own set of challenges, which once again I was unprepared for. For six months, every blood draw, every scan, and every infusion had to be done at City of Hope, four-hundred-plus miles from my home. Clinical drug trials follow strict protocols, so I ended up with something akin to a schedule, coordinated by the clinical trial nurse. Having a schedule comforted me (although because this is cancer we're talking about, the schedule was in constant flux).

I was often on a ridiculously early morning flight on the day of the appointment, or I flew down the night before, depending on the appointment time. Once I arrived at the airport I checked in with the special services desk (located next to the airline check-in desk area) and requested a wheelchair. I was pushed in a wheelchair through the airport (more on that later) and boarded the flight early. When we landed I either walked or had a wheelchair take me to the rental car agency. My travel chemo buddy, often my sister, would try to finagle a fun car (a red sports car rather than a beige sedan; I mean, why not?), and then we would head to the hotel or the hospital, depending on the type of appointment. We always stayed at the same hotel, and if my appointment was the next day, we would either collapse and order food or go out and grab a bite. If it was early we might get in our robes and watch bad television, or read, or I would do some writing. I can't say enough how much this routine meant to me; the front desk got to know us, and I always tried, often successfully, to get the same room. Don't be shy about requesting the same room or the same floor; if it makes you feel comfortable, it's one less thing to worry about. Just that little bit of familiarity—knowing the hotel, sleeping on the left side of the room—made the trips more bearable. Hotel chains often offer discounts for patients, either directly or through the hospital, so be sure to ask. I felt beyond lucky, obviously, to be part of the clinical trial, but leaving the kids every week broke my heart. So the routine helped take away the sting of it.

On the day of the appointment we woke up early, stopped at my favorite bakery for breakfast if I was allowed to eat, or got lunch food and sweets to bring with us to the hospital. By month two the staff at the café knew us and would wave or ask me how I was; it felt like having extra people on my team. These small rituals comforted me. The chemo trips started to feel like business trips; you might not want to be there, but it's your job and there's nothing to do but jump in with both feet and try to enjoy it.

We drove to the hospital, parked, and made sure we had the waiting-room bag of magazines, food, and water. After checking in with two different receptionists and getting a blood draw, we were given an estimated wait time. If the doctor or hospital was running three or more hours late, we turned back around, found the nearest movie theater, and sat in the cold air conditioning until it was time for the checkup or infusion.

Luckily, amazingly, we were able to pay for most of the flights, but friends and family generously gave airline miles for us to use as well. (If you're a member of any travel-related rewards program, or have points for airline flights, rental cars, or hotels, this is the time to use them.) I flew on commercial airlines, not knowing that there were resources available to cancer patients for travel; see Resources for more on travel support for cancer patients.

This is what kept me sane when traveling for, and during, treatment:

- Travel buddies. Whether it's one person who can go with you for every chemo trip or a rotating lineup of friends and family, make a list. You cannot travel alone if you are seriously ill. I took some flights alone when I felt stronger, but I always had someone waiting for me at either end. When selecting a buddy, keep in mind that the person needs to be able to deal with stress, boredom, and unexpected moments like a random bout of vomiting; hopefully they are funny, too. They must also be able to tolerate last-minute changes in plans and hours of waiting. Most importantly, this buddy will have to take detailed notes during the doctor appointments. Do not select anyone who will make the time seem to pass even more slowly or who will add to your anxiety or angst. (This might rule out family members and certain friends; this is okay.)

- Pack for two days even if you're scheduled to be gone for one day. A variety of things can go wrong, and believe me, it's better to have an extra pair of underwear, a toothbrush, and a fresh shirt than not. That said, you can usually find a Walmart, Target, or similar store near a hospital in case you need last-minute essentials. I bought many an emergency outfit at Target after an appointment ran long and we missed our flight, or my blood count was too low and I had to stay another night.

- Be sure to rent a car with GPS. You do not want to be driving around lost, stressing about being late to an appointment. Funny thing about the medical world: They keep you waiting, but you are not allowed to be late.

- Wash your hands constantly and carry hand sanitizer with you. Travel is a dirty business.

- You generally cannot take children under the age of fourteen with you into medical centers. Check the rules of your particular medical center, and be sure to check before making any plans. (Because kids come in contact with so many germs, they're generally not allowed around patients with compromised immune systems.) I didn't want my kids to come anyway, knowing how boring it would be and how horrible I would feel. But I did try to plan little family trips around the end of my chemo trips when I could, so depending on where your treatment is, that might be an option. (Folding in a visit to Disneyland with a chemo trip in Los Angeles, or a visit to Hersheypark if your treatment is at Penn State Hershey Medical Center in Hershey, Pennsylvania, for example, could make everyone happy.)

- Ask about disability access at amusement or theme parks, such as Disneyland. If you need special assistance or access, don't be embarrassed; ask at the ticket booth or guest services window. It will make the trip more enjoyable for everyone if you are comfortable and able to enjoy it.

- Take advantage of the help available to you for air travel. There are wheelchairs, early boarding, and several other options for passengers who are physically compromised. Don't be shy about asking for them. When you board the plane, for example, you can ask the flight attendant about getting a wheelchair upon your arrival. If you're in an airport with flights of steps and you have carry-on bags, there are back elevators available. Don't take the stairs just because you don't want to cause trouble; I did it once and almost passed out. Not worth it. You just have to make it happen.

- Pack something from home that comforts you. I always had a drawing from my daughter with me, or a little random stuffed animal or keychain she had stuck in my bag, and photos of my kids. Whatever it is, put it in your bag.

- Make a music playlist. I made a "Kick Cancer's Ass" playlist that my sister and I would blast on the way to the hospital, and it was kind of like the theme from the movie *Rocky* in the way that it would get me in a certain mind frame. Whether it's chanting, meditation, jazz, heavy metal, Beyoncé, or Taylor Swift, load it onto your mobile device and plug in.

- Expect the unexpected. Pack an extra magazine, or extra battery, or whatever you need in case the plane is delayed, or the doctor is delayed, or both.

- Most large medical centers have a patient or family room filled with books, couches, tables, and, most importantly, computers and printers. It's like a library; it's a quiet space to go in the middle of a beeping, frantic place. We used it on every visit to City of Hope to type up appointment notes, send out updates, and print out boarding passes. There is often a volunteer staffer who can answer questions, too.

PLANNING A GETAWAY:
A DAY OFF FROM CANCER

If you're planning a vacation during treatment, consider getting travel insurance in case you have to cancel at the last minute. Being a cancer patient means literally taking one day at a time, and you never know if your counts might be too low or if you'll react to a drug or spike a fever that could require you to stay home. Better to be safe than sorry. Even though many airlines, cruise lines, and hotels will credit or refund money with a letter from a doctor or hospital stating your inability to travel, travel insurance is one extra step.

If you are traveling alone or going abroad, it's wise to make a document that details your condition, recent treatment, medications, allergies, adverse reactions to drugs, and emergency contacts (both relatives and doctors). Pack two copies with you. If you are traveling to a place where you don't know the language, you might consider having your medical information translated to the local language, just in case of emergency. Also, pack all prescription medication in your carry-on luggage and bring copies of your prescriptions. If you have to take injections with syringes, bring instructions from your doctor in case you are stopped by airport personnel, at home or abroad. (I've been held up in airport security for simply wearing my compression sleeves.)

If you feel limited physically but want to travel for fun, pick a travel itinerary where you can be present but not be pushed beyond your limits. For example, instead of a walking trip around a city, visit somewhere with trains, tour buses, or trams where you can sit and look at the sights.

Just be realistic. If you are suffering and in treatment, it might not be the best time to take that trip to Morocco or climb Machu Pichu. Travel is exhausting even when you're in perfect health, and jet lag and packing and unpacking can take a toll. I understand the urge to flee, to see something new, to taste a new flavor when you're not sure there will be a next month or a next year. But don't put yourself (or your family) through a potentially disastrous trip if deep down you know you're not up to it.

Whether you're traveling for treatment or for rest and relaxation, there are a few other considerations to keep in mind.

Altitude: If your travel plans include any major changes in altitude, whether you're driving to the mountains or taking a flight, tell your doctor. Changes in altitude can have a major effect on cancer patients in terms of oxygen. (Check with the airline beforehand if you need to bring oxygen with you.) Altitude can also trigger lymphedema, so your doctor might recommend compression garments. These are available at specialty pharmacies and medical supply stores. They have to be fitted individually, which takes time, so plan accordingly. They are also usually covered by insurance. But sitting on long flights also increases the risk of blood clots (thrombosis), and patients undergoing chemotherapy or who have recently had surgery have a higher risk of clots. If you are traveling more than three hours by plane, get up every hour to get your circulation moving. (I carried a letter from my oncologist with me that explained my condition to show any flight attendant who was reluctant to let me roam the aisles.)

On the plane, drink bottled water and avoid ice to minimize exposure to germs.

Motion sickness might be an issue, whether you're traveling by car, bus, train, or plane. It's better to pack vomit bags than to be searching for them when it hits. Ordinary plastic bags (preferably in a color, not clear plastic) are good to pack, and there are also brands of motion sickness bags like Sic-Sac and CareBag, available at most drugstores if you want something "official."

MOVE IT:
EXERCISING DURING TREATMENT

"Keep moving" is the most important thing anyone said to me when I was diagnosed. I took it to heart, although that didn't mean I was up for any serious exercise at many points during treatment. Stretching your legs is part of any road trip.

Movement is a critical part of preventing side effects from treatment. Choose a safe activity and also one that will limit exposure to germs. For example, yoga may be a way to help you stretch, but bring your own yoga mat to avoid germs. A full round of golf may be off the table, but you might be able to go to a putting green and hit a few balls. If you can't train for a marathon, you might be able to jog around a local park. Even if you have to skip mountain biking, you can still possibly bike around a park or your neighborhood. Don't be stubborn about it; just because you can't do what you did before doesn't necessarily mean any movement is forbidden. (And hopefully this is just a temporary setback in your routine.) Just clear it with the doctors before you embark on any serious exercise program; they might have valid reasons for a specific exercise plan, or they could have other suggestions for you. You might have to adapt a type of exercise to your needs. But ultimately it's about finding something you will stick with. (For more on exercise, see Recurrence in chapter 12.)

CHAPTER 11

THE LANGUAGE OF CANCER: TALKING POINTS

The most hilarious, surreal moment for me as a patient was when an older relative referred to my cancer as "the Troubles." It became a family joke, and even now, before I go to an appointment, I tell my sister I'm leaving "to see the doctor about my Troubles." Because really, the whole thing is so absurd that you just have to laugh. I'm so grateful that I was sick in this time in history, when cancer patients aren't treated like pariahs or locked away in the back wards of hospitals, or during a time when ovarian cancer was referred to as "women's cancer" and breast cancer was called "women's disease." Cancer is treated with so much more consideration for our humanity, and a lot more awareness. But the flip side of all that openness and "open dialogue" is the things people say to you. (There might be moments when you long for the days when most people said nothing at all.)

Get ready for a few faux pas and more than one foot inserted squarely in mouth. I wish I had known to expect this, to create sort of a mental barrier to ward off any of the often wildly inappropriate things people said to me. Consider yourself warned.

OVERSHARING AND WHAT NOT TO SAY TO SOMEONE WITH CANCER

As a patient, you become acutely aware of everyone's words and actions. Sharing is good in theory—it creates a bond and is a form of trust—but sometimes family and friends overshare. For example, if you've looked up the patient's illness and possible survival rate, that is something to keep to yourself. If you know someone who died of a similar disease, don't share the news. Patients are often dealing with information overload, both from the medical side and from loved ones, and adding this kind of information to the mix isn't helpful.

What struck me as a cancer patient was the complete kindness as well as the complete lack of kindness. Total strangers reached out to me or comforted me in unexpected ways, but I'll never forget the people who stared at me, avoided my gaze, or wouldn't get near me. It was very hard to come to terms with. If you are visiting a cancer friend, take the time to ready yourself mentally and physically. They might look different, smell different, and act different. But don't give that away in your eyes or your actions. We patients already feel like strangers in our own bodies; we don't need reminding that we don't look like ourselves, too.

The Least Helpful Things to Say to a Cancer Patient

These are quotes of things that were said directly to me at various stages of my treatment and survivorship. Read, don't repeat!

- "Think of all the money you'll save in groceries!" (Referring to the number of meals dropped off by family, friends, and neighbors.)

- "This is the new normal."

- "Well, at least you get a new pair of boobs at the end of it."

- "You didn't want more kids anyway."

- "It's not the anesthesia you should be worried about—it's the surgery."

- "Oh, I know x or y; I looked up your cancer on the Internet."

- "My friend/sister/cousin/girlfriend/wife was diagnosed and now she is doing fine! You would never know!"

- "It must not have been as bad as they thought."

- "At least you don't have [fill in the blank] cancer here."

- "They do thousands of these [surgeries] a year."

- "How *are* you?" (Usually said with their forehead wrinkled and eyes wide.)

- "So you're done!" (Done with treatment. No, but thanks for asking.)

- "But you don't look sick."

- "I know too much." (From a friend who is in the world of breast cancer drug research and development.)

- "Are you just back from vacation?" (This from a friend who hadn't see me in a while, remarking on my radiation "tan.")

- "You look greeeaattt!"

- "Well, you're done now, and that's all behind you!"

HANDLE WITH CARE:
HOW TO TALK TO YOUR PATIENT—
A GUIDE FOR CARETAKERS

- Refrain from judgment. The word "shouldn't" is best avoided at all costs.

- Don't ask, "How are you?" unless you really want to hear the answer. Rephrasing is useful: "What are you feeling?" is more realistic and often easier to answer.

- Be patient. It's a frustrating thing to watch, but silence and crying are the norm. Try to understand that these emotions seemingly come and go.

- Be honest with the patient—to a point. If there are grand illusions, you might want to step in. But if the patient is talking about one day redecorating the living room or taking a trip to Tahiti, let them have their dreams! A little magical thinking is allowed.

- There isn't one right thing to say! Don't feel pressured to come up with something just to fill the silence.

- Help the patient with small goals: one day of getting through the pain or nausea or fatigue, then a week of getting through it, then a month. If you think or talk about the future too much it becomes too abstract. Small, achievable goals are better.

- Let the patient talk, and don't interrupt. Let them express their emotions, openly and without fear of what they sound like (scared, freaked out, furious, terrified).

- Your patient might need to grieve; this is a natural part of a cancer diagnosis. (For more on the stages of grief, see Navigating the River of Denial and Other Emotional Rollercoasters in chapter 3.)

- Try not to act tired/put upon/overwhelmed in front of the patient. It just causes more tension and guilt in an already-surreal situation. Leave the apartment or house, if you must—go for a walk around the block, or go to a friend's house to put your feet up and watch the game. (My favorite line relating to this: My survivor friend D., mother of two, who saw her husband lying on the couch one day while she was in treatment, said, "Oh, so you're having cancer today?" He got up and helped her.)

- Making up the bed with fresh sheets is often the best thing you can do (remember to use fragrance-free detergent). If a patient is spending a fair amount of time in bed sweating and feeling miserable, a set of cool, fresh sheets can make their day. (I called it "clean sheet day.")

Required Reading

When you feel like reading, you might want to be inspired by people who have been through it—*it* meaning a life-changing health issue, an unbelievable obstacle, or a seemingly impossible set of circumstances. These are books that I kept on my bedside table and returned to again and again.

- *Lucky Man: A Memoir* by Michael J. Fox

- *It's Always Something* by Gilda Radner

- *Life, on the Line: A Chef's Story of Chasing Greatness, Facing Death, and Redefining the Way We Eat* by Grant Achatz

- *Still Me* and *Nothing is Impossible: Reflections on a New Life* by Christopher Reeve

- *Survival Lessons* by Alice Hoffman

- *Unbroken: A World War II Story of Survival, Resilience, and Redemption* by Laura Hillenbrand

PART 3

SURVIVAL

CHAPTER 12

CLEAR MARGINS

SURVIVAL

Survival is complicated. But welcome to the club—according to the ACS, as of January 1, 2016 there were almost 16 million cancer survivors in the United States! You're suddenly, happily, pushed back into the world, but it's often not the same, and sometimes it's not even a world you recognize. People mean well and will pat you on the back and say, "You're done!" But it can be hard to return to everyday life after months or years of being deep in Cancerland. Your title changes, as well: One day you're a patient and the next day you're a survivor. The road trip is over but your heart is still on the open highway.

As a survivor, you're alive, but you often don't get a clean bill of health or hear the words "cured" or "done" or "remission" from the doctors. And because even the doctors usually can't or won't say exactly what the future will hold, you're stuck piecing together information and trying to look ahead without constantly worrying about a recurrence. My non-Hodgkin's lymphoma survivor friend looks at things this way: Every time she has a sore throat she thinks of the worst possible scenario, and she's five years clean. It's difficult not to live in fear, and that is something few people outside of the cancer circle understand. Getting comfortable in survivorship—or "thrivorship," as I like to say—can take time.

I often felt like I had landed back on the planet after a long time away, much like an astronaut would feel after a year on a space mission. You're back, and you recognize a few things, but you've been to places you can hardly describe to anyone else. I call it re-entry, and it may take longer than you anticipate.

FOLLOW-UP PLAN

Before you're "set free" back into the world, make another list of questions for your doctors. This will provide you with some sense of security that someone has your back, especially if you're worried about recurrence. Particularly if you have more than one doctor, it can be confusing to figure out which doctor prescribes which drug or whom to call if you have a medical question. After constant medical appointments and hovering medical professionals, it can be daunting to go months without an appointment. It's one of the ironies of cancer.

If your oncologist won't be your direct contact after treatment is completed, these are some questions to bring up at your last appointment with him or her:

- Which doctor do I see and when?

- Do I need to find a new GP (general practitioner) or PCP (primary care physician) who is familiar with the needs of cancer survivors?

- What follow-up tests do I need and when?

- Who will prescribe any medication that I have to take?

- Are there any symptoms I should watch for?

- Will insurance cover follow-up care?

POST-TRAUMATIC STRESS DISORDER (PTSD)

Most people think of PTSD as a war-related condition, triggered by extreme stress or trauma. But it's actually also a common condition for cancer survivors and their families. Technically it refers to a set of symptoms that develop after a stressful (often life-threatening) incident. The NCI refers to PTS as similar to, but not as severe as, PTSD. PTS can develop at any time during or after treatment. Symptoms like extreme anxiety, shock, reliving troubling events, having fearful thoughts, avoiding interaction with people, and insomnia are a few things to watch for. It's no wonder; cancer is nothing if not a set of repeated stresses. If you or someone you love is showing any of these symptoms of PTS, talk to the doctor and get a referral to a therapist or mental health specialist. PTS can be debilitating, particularly if the patient is already facing the stresses of illness and treatment. Treatment for PTS can include relaxation techniques like meditation, support groups, and medication. Depression, which affects 15 to 25 percent of cancer patients according to the NCI, can have similar symptoms.

The NCI found that "breast cancer survivors who had more advanced cancer or lengthy surgeries, or a history of trauma or anxiety disorders, were more likely" to be diagnosed with PTSD. Cancer recurrence can also be a factor in developing PTS. (Source: PDQ, Physician Data Query, NCI's database.) PTS is set off by "triggers"—certain memories that are sparked by sights or smells. I felt this acutely when I visited friends in hospitals; it was hard for me to sit in a vinyl chair and hear the beeping and smell the chemicals without reliving some of my own illness. I also couldn't go back to my mom's house, the place where I received my diagnosis, for almost six months. It was just too painful. The NCI notes that PTS generally shows symptoms about three months after the initial trauma but can also show itself years later, and that cancer survivors and their families should have long-term monitoring. Finding a mental health professional who is familiar with PTS and depression can be an important part of survivorship.

RECURRENCE

Fear of recurrence, or a return of cancer cells, is a reality for many survivors. It is understandable, but it doesn't have to dominate your life as a survivor. To quell your fears, ask your oncologist a few simple questions:

- What is my risk of recurrence?

- Is there anything I need to do to reduce my risk?

- How will I be monitored for recurrence?

The return back home after your road trip through Cancerland can be fraught with its own set of terms and considerations. A few that are vital to know:

Follow-up scans: These vary widely depending on the stage and type of cancer you have, but generally are scheduled every three months and then reduced to every six months and eventually yearly. The scans are generally CT, PET, or PET/CT combination scans. Some types of cancer require constant screening (blood tests or scans) or lifelong medication, while other patients require nothing but a yearly checkup. Being set free back into the world can feel liberating yet simultaneously terrifying; don't be surprised (or beat yourself up) if you have lasting paranoia about medical issues. This is perfectly normal. Anxiety among cancer survivors is common. The trick is to stay calm and have a good relationship with your oncologist so they can calm you down and discuss your concerns.

Lifestyle changes: As a survivor, you may need to gain, lose, or maintain weight. Some studies have shown that cancer survivors often have poor diets or are overweight. Getting or staying in shape is not just about fitting into a pair of pants; excess weight can cause your body to produce excess hormones and affect molecules that can make tumors grow. Exercise is key for survivors! Getting the HHS's recommended one hundred fifty minutes of moderate to vigorous exercise every week is one standard, but ask your oncologist what they recommend for your specific case. I make a daily thirty-minute walk part of my survivorship—it is a non-negotiable part of my day. If you can't walk in your neighborhood, there might be resources available through the hospital or in your community, such as a physical therapist covered by your insurance. Some gyms offer free week-long passes, and some offer reduced-rate memberships to cancer patients (a letter from your oncologist is usually all you need to bring). Or maybe there is a personal trainer that works on a sliding scale who could teach you some basic exercises to replicate at home. If you want to swim or do water fitness classes, research public pools in your area. They might have discounts for cancer patients and survivors or offer reduced rates. Exercise comes in many forms: Dance classes, yoga, or Pilates might be the right fit for you. There might even be a local basketball, soft-ball, or adult soccer league in your community. Once again, a little research can yield big results. TeamSurvivor (team-survivor.org) is a nonprofit with affiliates in many cities and regions throughout the United States that focuses on group fitness programs for female cancer survivors; go to their web-site to search for a program in your zip code. WeCanRow, a program run by Camp Randall Rowing Club in Madison, Wisconsin, offers female cancer survivors rowing and fitness training. And "Livestrong at the YMCA" offers twelve-week fitness programs for cancer survivors at four-hundred loca-tions in the United States; check Livestrong.org for a loca-tion. Find something you like and get moving.

Creating and sticking with the wellness plan that works for you might require consulting a nutritionist or dietician or talking to a professional about creating an exercise program. Many medical centers offer wellness programs with reduced fees to access nutrition, physical, and mental health professionals. Be sure to ask your doctor or nurse about programs at your medical center. Your health insurance company or your employer might also offer exercise programs.

Often word of mouth can also get you further than you think; your kid's science teacher might know of a martial arts studio with night classes, or your sister's coworker might have a background in personal training. The old cliché "ask and you shall receive" is worth trying. Think outside the box and don't be afraid to ask. There are probably more resources available in your community than you think. The worst thing that can happen is that people say no; and really, haven't you already been through the worst thing?

Follow-up surgeries: Planning for any follow-up surgeries is also part of survivorship. If you're a breast cancer patient who has undergone breast reconstruction, talk to your plastic surgeon about any follow-up care and any symptoms to watch for. (Breast implants can be finicky, and some women require two or three surgeries to get them right.) Some types of implants have to be replaced periodically; this is important to keep in mind. (See chapter 4 for more information.)

Osteoporosis: another word for bone loss. Cancer treatment can take a toll on bones.

We lose bone mass as we age, but younger cancer patients can experience it much earlier due to certain treatments, including chemotherapy and radiation. Osteoporosis occurs when the cells that rebuild bone don't get replaced as quickly as they die, causing brittle, thin bones. A bone mineral density (BMD) test—a painless, low-dose X-ray—is used to establish a baseline, then treatment can be prescribed, whether it's increased doses of calcium or, in extreme cases, medications. (The test is usually covered by health insurance.)

Hormone replacement therapy (also referred to as HRT or HT): HRT has been a controversial therapy for female cancer patients. Prescribing hormones (estrogen and progestin) to menopausal women to ease symptoms like hot flashes and possibly prevent osteoporosis began in the 1990s. In 2002, however, the Women's Health Initiative (WHI) published results of a long-term study questioning the use of these hormones and raised the issue of the risks involved (heart attacks, breast cancer, and stroke, for example).

Hormone therapy is used in both pre- and post-menopausal women and can be given before, during, or after other forms of cancer treatment. It can be used as an adjuvant therapy or neoadjuvant therapy (see Cancerspeak, Part 2, in chapter 2 for these definitions). Hormone medications come in tablet form, with the exception of Faslodex (fulvestrant), which is given by injection in a doctor's office.

There are myriad factors that go into deciding your hormone therapy regimen, including history of blood clots, risk of uterine or ovarian cancer, and the stage of breast cancer. You might start taking one medication and then be switched to another type years later, depending on your specific type of breast cancer. On average, breast cancer patients take some form of hormone medicine for five years.

There are three types of hormonal therapy medications:

- Aromatase inhibitor (AI): AI medications block the production of estrogen. Letrozole (a.k.a. Femara) is a common type.

- Selective estrogen receptor modulator (SERM): Tamoxifen is the most well-known. A newer chemotherapy drug that is similar to tamoxifen is called exemestane; see the NCI website for more info. (See Cancerspeak, Part 2, in chapter 2 for more on tamoxifen.)

- Estrogen receptor downregulator (ERD): Faslodex (fulvestrant) is the most common.

This is just a brief introduction to a complicated and somewhat controversial topic that you can discuss with your oncologist and/or gynecologist.

Lymphedema: If you've been treated for breast cancer, you have to watch for signs of lymphedema. (The risk of lymphedema depends on the type of treatment; breast cancer patients who have had both surgery and radiation are at higher risk.) Besides breast cancer, lymphedema can develop in any cancer patient who has had radiation or surgery involving the head, neck, pelvis, or groin.

Lymph nodes are pea-sized pieces of tissue that make up the lymphatic system. Lymph nodes and vessels collect and carry lymph fluid (which contains proteins, white blood cells, salts, and water) through the body. When a lymph node is surgically removed, the lymph vessels are removed as well, and that changes the flow of lymph fluid in that side of the body. (In some cases, lymph nodes are removed from both sides of the body.) When the flow changes, the remaining nodes and vessels work overtime, and if they can't get rid of the fluid, it builds up and causes swelling. The swelling occurs in your arms or legs and can feel like a tightening sensation; it is one symptom of lymphedema. Lymphedema usually develops slowly over time and can occur months or even years after radiation or surgery.

The trick with lymphedema is that it is untreatable, so prevention is key. If you've had surgery, the surgeon should go over lymphedema symptoms and prevention, and if you've had radiation therapy the radiation oncologist should review the risks with you. But there are many do's and don'ts for lymphedema prevention, so make an appointment to go over the details.

Living with the risk of lymphedema is another thing I had to add to my list. It changed the way I exercise, travel, and even go grocery shopping (I can't lift bags of groceries anymore). Making adjustments and using workarounds (like grocery delivery) is how I've approached it (with just a little bit of complaining on the side).

Creative Thank-You Notes

Writing thank-you cards by hand to every person who helped you along the road trip can seem overwhelming, particularly if the road trip has been going on for more than a year. Here are a few ways to show your gratitude that are more creative (and might be less exhausting for you) than taking pen to paper:

- Create photo postcards with a photo of you during or after treatment, or with friends or family (or pets!).

- Ask your kid(s) to draw a picture or make a card that you can photocopy and mail to your "support team."

- Write one thank-you card, scan it, and email it to your community if you want to skip the envelopes and postage.

- If you're a baker or home cook, make batches of your favorite spice mix or favorite cookie. Bag them up, tie them with a pretty ribbon, and drop them off at friends' and neighbors' houses. (If you can't drive, walk or ask your partner or spouse to drive you!)

- Make a donation to your favorite charity in the name of all who helped you.

- Don't forget to thank your medical team! Send a card to the medical office, hospital, lab, treatment center—wherever you received treatment—with a note of appreciation. (I still send holiday cards to every doctor and nurse I met on my road trip. I like to show them that I'm alive and oh-so grateful!)

HOT FLASHES AND MOOD SWINGS: HORMONES AND MENOPAUSE

Just when I thought I had enough going on—cancer, and then the side effects of treatment—I had to face the big M: menopause. For women dealing with a gynecological cancer diagnosis, a common side effect is immediate menopause. Surgically induced menopause is similar; this is defined as menopause that is triggered by the removal of the ovaries (oophorectomy) or the uterus (hysterectomy)—or both—which reduces the amount of estrogen and progesterone in the body. The ovaries contain eggs that secrete these two hormones that tumors need to grow, so removing the ovaries can slow down or eliminate the chance that these tumors will develop. (Sometimes fallopian tubes are removed as well—which is called a salpingo-oophorectomy.) But estrogen, which is only secreted through ovaries, also helps build bones, so women who undergo the surgery are at higher risk of broken bones.

Facing another set of side effects made me want to hide in the closet. Going into menopause can bring hot flashes, insomnia, night sweats, weight gain, mood swings, growth of facial hair, decreased sex drive, and vaginal dryness. Make an appointment with your gynecologist to discuss the symptoms; there might be a solution other than suffering through it. For example, a medication called venlafaxine (Effexor) can treat extreme hot flashes. Menopause naturally lasts an average of five to eight years, but if you're launched into it early, it can last anywhere from three to ten years.

For symptoms that are less dire but just as irritating, like facial hair, it's all a matter of hormones. The coarse hairs that appear on your chin and face are called terminal hairs and are caused by the menopausal imbalance of estrogen and testosterone (estrogen drops, testosterone keeps being produced). There is a prescription topical cream available to control facial hair growth, or you can take the non-medical route of waxing, tweezing, or electrolysis.

PILLOW TALK

Vaginal dryness and vaginal atrophy are common symptoms for women after chemo, radiation, and surgery for gynecological cancers or even cancers in the lower regions of the body such as the gallbladder. This can impact your sex life and even your everyday life. (That's one part of survivorship—you might actually think about having sex again!) And even the skin of the vagina itself, which thins as women age, can be affected by chemo and menopause. There's even a term for painful sex after menopause: dyspareunia.

Survivors often don't mention these lingering side effects—it's not exactly dinner-table conversation—but again, there might be a treatment out there. There has been debate in the medical community about the use of estrogen products in cancer patients and survivors, so there is a lot of information available. Products containing estrogen release a small amount, and only a small amount is absorbed into the bloodstream; side effects can include vaginal bleeding, breast pain, and nausea. Bring it up with your oncologist, but here are a few products to ask about:

- Vaginal estrogen cream: The cream essentially rebuilds the lining of the vagina and urethra by promoting collagen production. It usually works within three weeks. It can also be used for dryness and irritation on the outside of the vagina. Premarin and Estrace are common brand names.

- Vaginal estrogen ring: The ring is inserted into the vagina by the patient. Two common brand names are Estring and Femring.

- Vaginal tablet: This is inserted into the vagina twice a week by the patient. A common brand name is Vagifem.

- Osphena: This is an estrogen-free prescription medication that comes in tablet form. The medication acts like estrogen in the vagina, providing ongoing moisture.

Over-the-counter, non-prescription options that can be helpful for sexual intercourse are lubricants such as Luvena and Replens. They are both estrogen-free, but Luvena is glycerin- and paraben-free as well. (K-Y and Yes are also common brands.) Pure coconut or almond oil are also options, but be mindful when using oils that you keep them completely sanitary: You must wash your hands or use gloves to be sure no bacteria gets in the bottle.

Vaginal physical therapy: This may sound unusual, but there are physical therapists who work with women to recover sensation in their vaginas using non-medication based techniques. Ask your doctor for a recommendation; it might be covered by your health insurance plan.

And be sure to talk to your oncologist about birth control. It's possible to get pregnant (and impregnate) during treatment, which might not be ideal for either you (the patient) and/or the fetus for a variety of reasons. Whether you're in treatment or a survivor and you're sexually active, make sure you take precautions that you've cleared with your doctor!

It's very common for cancer patients and survivors to have physical and emotional issues around sex. Getting your "groove" back, for both female and male cancer patients (men who've gone through testicular, prostate, or lower-body cancer can face similar sexual dysfunction), can be a big issue. Feeling unattractive or uncomfortable with the "new you" is common, particularly for patients who have undergone surgery and are physically different than they were. You might not enjoy the same things that you used to, but that doesn't mean there aren't other ways to be intimate. Start small: You might start the trip back to the bedroom by buying new underwear, pajamas, or lingerie that make you feel sexy and scheduling some alone time with your partner. If you don't feel comfortable talking to your partner about your feelings about sex, find someone you can talk to. It can be extremely isolating and frustrating, and finding another survivor (or a doctor or a therapist) who understands can be comforting. Some cancer centers offer sexual health seminars or programs for survivors. If you're single and dating after treatment, considering intimacy with a new partner and discussing your health—Why is your hair short? What is that scar?—can seem overwhelming. Think about what you will or won't share with them. (This is where survivor groups can be extremely helpful; you can swap tips, advice, and stories without fear of judgment.) Talk, vent, communicate: The key with an often-ignored topic such as sex is to open up and be honest (for more about sex, see Cancer and Marriage in chapter 9).

Whether you're single or in a committed relationship, don't minimize your feelings on the topic of sex; these are real, valid emotions, and they are part of your life as both a patient and survivor.

MEET AND GREET: MEETING OTHER SURVIVORS

If you didn't get a chance to meet other cancer patients while you were busy on your own road trip, this can be the perfect time to reach out. There are survivor groups for every type of cancer and every age group. Participating in fundraisers is one way to meet survivors (and patients) in your area, but it doesn't mean you have to run a marathon to connect; survivors get together in every way imaginable. I met a woman who had met a group of breast cancer survivors through the Mana'olana Pink Paddlers in Maui, Hawaii; they paddle together in outrigger canoes twice a week and welcome all cancer survivors to participate. I heard about a nonprofit in my county (To Celebrate Life, www.tocelebratelife.org) that holds a fashion show fundraiser every year featuring breast cancer patients and survivors as models. I found out about it through a nurse, and I applied online. I was slightly anxious about dressing up and walking down a runway in high heels under bright lights, but I met the most incredible group of women and found friends that are now friends for life. It was truly one of the most amazing events of my life. We practiced every weekend for six weeks for the big night. There we were, young, old, bald, and with hair, all shapes and sizes—every single one of us smiling, strutting, and bursting with life as three hundred audience members cheered us on. I never thought I could feel pretty again, and it was a turning point in my survivorship.

If you feel up to it (mentally and physically), volunteering with a cancer-related nonprofit, program, or hospital can be a great use of your experience and time. There are so many programs that need volunteers, everything from knitting hats for patients and delivering meals to getting your dog certified as a therapy dog and bringing him into medical center waiting rooms. Now that you've seen what patients need, you might recognize friends or people around you who need advice, someone to sit with them, or someone to watch their kids for a couple of hours. You know how to be useful.

EXPECT THE UNEXPECTED

Be prepared to go crazy—or not! I took tap dance lessons, I galloped a horse faster than I should have, I gave a speech to two hundred people, I learned how to throw a baseball, I swam in the Mediterranean Sea. Some survivor friends run marathons, take up painting, take their dream trip to Alaska, or Mexico, or Fiji; some rearrange their whole lives. Some people relocate, some switch jobs or careers, some renew their marriage vows, while others file for divorce. Don't be surprised if this thing—this cancer road trip—leads to places you never could have imagined.

The craziest thing I did after I completed the trifecta (infusions, surgery, and radiation) was get a puppy! My best friend from high school and I drove two hours to pick up this eight-pound black-and-white ball of love. My husband and I had talked about getting a Dalmatian, and then when I got a call about a puppy, I was in. Tango is pure joy and gets me (and the whole family) outside and active. As writer (and survivor) Alice Hoffman says in her brilliantly poignant book *Survival Lessons*, "A puppy is never a mistake, though it is often a mess." Enough said.

PART 4

EPILOGUE

As of June 2016, I am living life! I'm a survivor, thriver, mom, wife, daughter, sister, friend. I am grateful, and I am fearless (within reason). I'm kinder in the grocery store line. And I say yes to more (and no to other stuff). I leave more days on the calendar empty, ready for spontaneity. I don't put things away to wait for a better time or the "right" time. This is the time.

Medically, I am thrilled to say that I came off the clinical trial chemotherapy drug in May 2015; my oncologist recommended I stop taking it due to possible long-term side effects (like a secondary cancer). I remain on hormone therapy, and I see my oncologist every three months for blood work and have scans every six months; the scans continue to show no sign of cancer.

I use the time I have more wisely; less time allotted to cleaning a cluttered garage and more time stomping in puddles with the kids and building fairy houses in the backyard. I've come to be at peace with the fact that we don't know—won't ever know, really—if cancer will come back into my life, but I do know I have the most amazing oncologist who is ready should I ever need him again. (And an update on the clinical trial drug Veliparib: It has moved forward to Phase III testing and is being studied on more than a dozen different types of cancers. It will hopefully be as effective for other cancer patients as it was for me and make it to market. I'm watching and waiting.)

Returning to life as a mom was incredible and something I viewed as a reintroduction. I had missed so many months of my son's toddler life, and it took a while for us to get to know each other. My daughter still asks me when I will grow my hair back to "normal" and when I will stop taking my pills. But I've developed better answers over time.

And it took me longer than I thought to adjust and embrace my physical life No more handstands in yoga, but I can hike and chase my dog. I can't carry my kids, but I can hold their hands. I can help pick out the pumpkins at Halloween, but I can't pick them up. It was, and sometimes still is, hard not to look back. It's hard to think about the "old" life—a life without pills, a life without pain and daily naps—but also hard not to constantly look over my shoulder to see if cancer is there, creeping up. Every ache, any bump or strange thing on my body has to be checked just to be sure. And that's a new feeling.

The depth of gratitude I feel every day is impossible to describe. I'm trying to pay it forward to other patients, to help ease some angst, to comfort. And to use my precious time to teach my kids about the world, to live, to give, and to do the Happy Dance whenever possible.

The Highest Highs, and the Lowest Lows

From the day of diagnosis onward, a few of my highs and lows:

High: My daughter saying: "You are a one and only."

High: Watching the sunset over the Pacific Ocean while sipping bubbly water next to my daughter.

High: When a gas-station cashier in Los Angeles bought me a lottery ticket because I "could use it."

High: Realizing that a lot of people were and are working very hard to keep me alive.

High: Rolling up my jeans and running away from the waves at the beach.

High: Finding three perfect sand dollars at the beach on my thirty-ninth birthday.

High: Feeling the wind blow through the few strands of hair that were growing back after chemo.

High: Kissing my children goodnight.

High: Getting the keys from the realtor to our first house, which we bought a couple of months after I finished radiation treatment.

High: Watching (and sobbing) while my sister showed a video montage she had made of my first "cancerversary."

High: Honoring my oncologist with a hospital award and getting a chance to thank him in front of his colleagues.

Low: Realizing that every minute does count.

Low: Cutting my finger while slicing an avocado and getting five stitches right in the middle of treatment. I drove myself to the local hospital with my finger wrapped in paper towels. Lying on the gurney in the emergency room trying to piece together my medical history to the attending physician was one of the longest hours of the entire "journey."

Low: Getting the stomach flu after chemo and throwing up in an indoor parking lot.

Low: Having our house robbed (and my husband's family heirlooms stolen) while I was away getting chemo.

Low: Thinking about someone other than me being called "Mommy."

Low: Kissing my kids goodnight on the nights before my surgeries.

Low: Watching the nurse unwrap the bandages after my double mastectomy.

Low: Having our car stolen from our front driveway. With the kids' car seats and my disabled parking placard in it.

Low: Having a totally inept nurse try to insert a catheter in dim lighting at 1:00 AM after my thirteen-hour surgery. (I told him to give it up and send in a female nurse.)

Record your highs and lows:

_____

_____

_____

_____

_____

_____

_____

_____

_____

_____

_____

_____

_____

_____

_____

_____

_____

_____

_____

_____

_____

MORNING (~7 AM)	# OF PILLS	FORM	MON 00/00/00 TAKEN?	TUES 00/00/00	WED 00/00/00	THURS 00/00/00	FRI 00/00/00	SAT 00/00/00	SUN 00/00/00
Drug Name (brand name & generic)	2	Tablets							
Ondanestron (Zofran)	1	Capsule							
Drug Name	1	Tablet							
DURING THE DAY (~2 PM)									
Drug Name									
Drug Name									
OPTIONAL (can be taken during the day)									
Drug Name									
Drug Name									
EVENING (~8 or 9 PM)									
Drug Name									
Drug Name									
Drug Name									

PART 5

NOTES

SAMPLE MEDICATION CHART

This is a sample chart (left) that you can use to create your own system for tracking medications. Whatever system you use, be sure to include the following information for each medication: name (brand name and generic, if applicable); dosage (amount in milligrams as well as time of day it should be taken); color of the pill or liquid; any drug interactions; date you began taking it; and why you're taking it.

SAMPLE QUESTIONS FOR YOUR ONCOLOGIST

While every type of cancer will require a specific set of questions, here are some general sample questions that you should ask the oncologist. When you're developing your own questions to add to this list, think of who, what, when, and how.

- What kind of tests will be performed and what do they tell me? And when can I expect the results?

- What are my treatment options? Do you have access to advanced treatment options, such as clinical drug trials?

- What are the side effects of treatment?

- How many patients have you treated with this type of cancer?

- How will you and your office help me navigate my treatment, including financial and insurance issues, medical resources or alternative therapies available through the office or medical center, and psychosocial or oncology-social worker resources?

- Does your office/medical center use a secure email system, or do we communicate by phone? If there is an email system, how do I set up the account, and how does it work?

- Where will I be treated?

- Who will be on my "team"—specialists, nurses? Who is my direct contact? Who is the after-hours contact?

- How are medication prescriptions handled? Is there a refill telephone line?

SAMPLE PATIENT "CHEAT SHEET"

Full name: _____

Date of birth: _____

Medical record number (MRN) (if applicable): _____

Medical insurance plan and plan number (and a contact phone number, if applicable): _____

_____

Allergies (drug allergies or other allergies, such as food):

_____

_____

Any known adverse reactions to any drugs: _____

_____

Medications (prescription and over-the-counter, including vitamins, supplements, etc.): _____

_____

Blood type: _____

Usual blood pressure reading, if available: _____

Primary care physician, with contact information:

_____

Other physician(s) consulted, with contact information:

_____

_____

Hospitalizations (where/when/reason): _____

_____

_____

Surgeries (where/when/reason): _____

_____

_____

For women: Date of last menstrual period: _____

For women: History of pregnancies and births: _____

_____

_____

Family history of illness: _____

_____

_____

Emergency contact (name and phone number):

_____

Advance medical directive (AMD) on file? _____

RESOURCES

There are myriad resources for cancer patients in the United States, available through both public and private organizations. It's just a matter of finding them. (This is the time to use the Internet—for resources as well as to help plan logistics.) Even the most obscure, rare cancers have foundations and supporters.

I've listed as many resources as I could here, but I highly encourage you and your "team" to research anything you might need—from a family retreat or survivor's hiking trip to finding assistance with the cost of a wig or prescription medication.

Because I am a breast cancer patient, there are a few more resources listed here that are dedicated to that specific cancer. But unless noted, the resources here are for all adult cancer patients, male and female.

General Services and National Organizations

American Brain Tumor Association: www.abta.org; (800) 886-2282
The ABTA is a national organization that funds brain tumor research as well as providing educational materials and resources to patients and caregivers.

American Cancer Society (ACS): www.cancer.org; (800) 227-2345
This is a national nonprofit that provides a wide range of assistance, from cancer facts and medical research to patient support, fundraisers, and events throughout the United States. The website is available in English,

Spanish, and several Asian languages. You can also have a live chat with an ACS representative and/or look for a local ACS office in your area. ACS also runs the tlc (Tender Loving Care) program, which sells hair-loss and mastectomy products such as wigs and breast prosthetics. TLC (Tender Loving Care): www.tlcdirect.org, (800) 850-9445

American Lung Association: www.lung.org; (800) 586-4872
This national nonprofit provides information, educational materials, and advocacy for lung health and diseases. They also provide specific resources for lung cancer patients, including an "action guide," a survivor support community, and "LungForce" program where patients and survivors can share their stories. Website also available in Spanish.

American Society of Clinical Oncology (ASCO):
www.asco.org, www.cancer.net
ASCO is a membership of oncologists, founded in 1964, that provides professional guidelines and advocacy for research, among other topics. Their patient-oriented website, www.cancer.net, provides reliable, detailed information about current cancer research, clinical drug trials, and tools for navigating cancer and survivorship. (Cancer.net is also available as a mobile app.)

American Thyroid Association: www.thyroid.org; (800) 849-7643
The ATA is a nonprofit that is devoted to prevention, research, and providing information about thyroid diseases, including educational materials about, and treatment guidelines for, thyroid cancer. (Thyroid cancer is a common cancer among young adults ages twenty to thirty-nine.) Educational materials also available in Spanish.

Association of Oncology Social Work (AOSW):
www.aosw.org, (847) 686-2233
AOSW is an international organization of oncology social workers. Their website offers a list of resources, a blog that covers patient issues, and tips for patients.

Be the Match: www.bethematch.org; (800) 627-7692
A nonprofit that provides extensive patient services and resources for blood cancer patients, including "Be the Match Registry," operated by the National Marrow Donor Program (NMDP) that matches patients with bone marrow and cord blood donors. Educational materials also available in Spanish.

CancerForward: www.cancerforward.org; (713) 840-0988
"The Foundation for Cancer Survivors," CancerForward is a nonprofit devoted to cancer survivorship, with resources, online support groups for cancer survivors of all ages. Started by a breast cancer survivor in Houston in 2010, the website provides helpful links to survivorship issues.

Cancer Support Community:
www.cancersupportcommunity.org, (888) 793-9355
This nonprofit provides a global network of assistance for cancer patients, from how to talk to your kids about cancer, clinical trials, and educational brochures on cancer topics ("Frankly Speaking About") to live chats. (This organization formed with the merger of The Wellness Community and Gilda's Club Worldwide.)

Dear Jack Foundation: www.dearjackfoundation.org
Founded by musician and leukemia survivor Andrew McMahon, Dear Jack is a nonprofit that offers programs, grants, and resources for young adult cancer patients and survivors (ages eighteen to thirty-nine). Their "LifeList" program helps fulfill a wish for a patient, from a visit to the set of a television show to a play structure for their kids, Dear Jack aims to make each patient's "LifeList" come true. The "Breathe Now" meet-up yoga program will launch in several cities throughout the United States, with the goal of introducing yoga, breath work, and meditation to patients and survivors.

Lacuna Loft: www.lacunaloft.org
A web-based nonprofit founded by a Hodgkin's lymphoma survivor that "provides young adult cancer resources no matter where you are."

They offer a range of online support for patients, survivors, and caregivers ages eighteen to thirty-nine. Their goal is to end the isolation that is common among cancer patients; info on topics like dating and sex during treatment, exercise, and nutrition are available as well as a book club, journaling group, and writing group.

Leukemia & Lymphoma Society: www.lls.org; (914) 949-5213
A national nonprofit with local chapters, the LLS is dedicated to "fighting blood cancers." They provide detailed educational information about blood cancers in addition to offering resources such as peer-to-peer support for patients and caregivers. The LLS website is also available in Spanish.

National Cancer Information Center: (800) 227-2345
Run by the American Cancer Society, this center is available for patient information twenty-four hours a day, seven days a week; Spanish and other language assistance is also available.

National Cancer Institute (NCI):
www.cancer.gov, (800) 4-CANCER (1-800-422-6237)
This is an extremely helpful resource for medical explanations and finding cancer care; online chat help is also available.

The National Hospice and Palliative Care Organization:
www.nhpco.org, (800) 658-8898
An organization that provides detailed resources, education, and support for patients facing end-of-life and end-of-care decisions.

National Institutes of Health (NIH): www.nih.gov
NIH oversees the NCI and CDC. It also has a small clinical practice where they treat some patients with rare cancers as part of a study at their facility in Bethesda, Maryland. Another good source for clinical trial listings.

National LGBT Cancer Network: www.cancer-network.org
This program advocates for, and provides resources to, lesbian, gay, bisexual, and transgender cancer patients.

Nueva Vida: www.nueva-vida.org; (202) 223-9100
This is a nonprofit dedicated to helping Latinos and Latinas through the entire cancer process, from diagnosis to survivorship. They have three offices to serve patients in the mid-Atlantic states: Baltimore, Washington, DC, and Richmond, Virginia. Education materials are available in both English and Spanish, and the website is available in Spanish.

Oral Cancer Foundation:
www.oralcancerfoundation.org, (949) 723-4400
Founded by oral cancer survivor Brian Hill, the OCF was set up to educate the public about oral cancer as well as provide patients with educational resources such as financial assistance, health insurance information, and clinical trial listings. In addition to funding oral cancer research and patient advocacy, the website offers a secure patient online chat forum for oral cancer patients.

Stupid Cancer: www.stupidcancer.org; (877) 735-4673
This nonprofit, founded by a young adult brain cancer survivor, is devoted to the young adult cancer population (ages eighteen to thirty-nine). Based in New York City, they offer a wide variety of services, resources, and events for patients and survivors.

Testicular Cancer Society:
www.testicularcancersociety.org, (513) 696-9827
Founded by a testicular cancer survivor in Ohio, TCS provides support and resources for men diagnosed with testicular cancer (which is the leading type of cancer among men ages fifteen to thirty-five).

The Ulman Cancer Fund for Young Adults (UCF):
www.ulmanfund.org, (888) 393-3863
This Baltimore nonprofit was created by a survivor for cancer patients and survivors who are fifteen to thirty-nine years old. The UCF offers a variety of support services, including peer connections, college schol-arships for patients and survivors, patient navigation support, exercise

support for survivors, and direct support for patients being treated in Maryland and the Washington, DC, area.

US Food and Drug Administration (FDA):
www.fda.gov, (855) 543-3784
The FDA is a reliable source for information about drugs and medical devices, from side effects and medicine safety to clinical trials and drug approvals. They also have information about safely disposing of medications. (The FDA falls under HHS, Department of Health and Human Services.)

Financial Information/Counseling and Legal and Employment Resources

CancerCare: www.cancercare.org; (800) 813-4673
CancerCare is a national organization that offers financial assistance programs for people affected by cancer and provides publications and other resources, including the AVONCares direct financial assistance program for breast cancer patients.

The Cancer Financial Assistance Coalition (CFAC):
www.cancerfac.org
CFAC is a group of national organizations that provide financial help to patients. The group offers a national database of financial resources that's searchable by both diagnosis and type of resource needed.

Cancer for College: www.cancerforcollege.org; (760) 599-5096
A nonprofit started by two-time cancer survivor and amputee Craig Pollard, Cancer for College provides scholarships for cancer survivors and amputees of all ages enrolled in a college in the United States and Puerto Rico. Apply online.

Cancer Legal Resource Center:
www.disabilityrightslegalcenter.org/cancer-legal-resource-center,
(866) THE-CLRC (1-866-843-2572)
Part of the Disability Rights Legal Center in Los Angeles, the CLRC provides information and education about insurance, employment, and other cancer-related legal issues to both cancer patients and healthcare professionals.

Cancer + Careers: www.cancerandcareers.org
This is a nonprofit that helps cancer patients in the workplace, including providing educational materials, seminars, and career coaching.

Equal Employment Opportunity Commission (EEOC): www.eeoc.gov, (800) 669-4000
The EEOC website has information about cancer in the workplace in terms of employee and employer rights. (The website is also available in Spanish and six other languages.) They also have fifteen district offices that can be contacted.

GiveForward: www.giveforward.com
With GiveForward, individuals can create a free web page to request funding assistance, and it includes a specific section for fundraising for cancer patients and medical bills. They charge an average fee of 5 percent to process payments.

HealthWell Foundation: www.healthwellfoundation.org, (800) 675-8416
This independent nonprofit organization helps patients with chronic, life-altering diseases pay for deductibles, insurance premiums, and medication costs. There are certain exceptions, so check the website.

HOPE for Young Adults with Cancer: www.hope4yawc.org
This nonprofit helps young adult cancer patients ages eighteen to forty with financial assistance, special events, resource navigation, and information.

National Foundation for Transplants (NFT): www.transplants.org, (800) 489-3863
NFT provides funds for patients needing transplants, including bone marrow and stem cell transplants.

National Society of Genetic Counselors (NSGC): www.nsgc.org
NSGC provides a list of genetic counselors in the United States.

Ralph Lauren Center for Cancer Care:
www.ralphlaurencenter.org, (212) 987-1777

Working in partnership with Memorial Sloan Kettering Hospital in New York City, the Ralph Lauren Center provides referrals as well as services like dental care, psychotherapy, legal services, and Care Navigators, who coordinate with nurses and staff to help patients navigate cancer from diagnosis through survivorship. Currently the Center works with patients in every borough in New York City. They accept many insurance plans and also have a financial assistance program for qualified patients. Appointments are available through their website or by phone.

Medication and Treatment Assistance

The Assistance Fund: theassistancefund.org; (855) 845-3663

The Assistance Fund provides financial support to chronically ill patients with high-cost medications.

Good Days: www.mygooddays.org

Good Days helps patients with a chronic disease pay health insurance co-pays for medication.

National Patient Advocate Foundation (PAF): www.npaf.org

NPAF helps patients work with insurers, employers, and those to whom they owe medical debt, and can often help patients who are denied access to clinical drug trials or denied coverage for prescription drugs.

NeedyMeds: www.needymeds.org; (800) 503-6897

This is an information source about companies that offer patient assistance programs, which help those who cannot afford medications obtain them through the manufacturer at no or low cost.

Partnership for Prescription Assistance:
www.pparx.org, (888) 477-2669

This program helps qualified patients who lack prescription drug coverage obtain the medications they need through patient assistance programs.

Patient Access Network (PAN) Foundation:
www.panfoundation.org, (866) 316-7263
The PAN Foundation assists cancer patients with out-of-pocket costs associated with their treatment.

Patient Services, Inc. (PSI):
www.patientservicesinc.org, (800) 366-7741
PSI provides assistance with health insurance premiums, co-payments, and travel expenses for people with chronic diseases. Apply online.

PfizerRxPathways: www.pfizerrxpathways.com; (866) 706-2400
A patient assistance program from Pfizer, a pharmaceutical company. The program helps eligible patient get access to Pfizer medicine at a discount or for free; they also provide insurance counseling and co-pay assistance. They work with health clinics and hospitals in every state with a searchable database by zip code. Apply online; website is also available in Spanish.

RxHope: rxhope.com; (877) 267-0517
RxHope helps cancer patients obtain free or low-cost prescription medications.

StudyConnect: www.BMSStudyConnect.com; (855) 907-3286
This website is run by Bristol-Meyers Squibb (BMS), a biopharmaceutical company, and provides information about clinical studies sponsored by BMS.

Resources for Parents in Treatment
American Academy of Child and Adolescent Psychiatry (AACAP), aacap.org
A professional organization of child and adolescent psychiatrists, their website includes information to help families talk about cancer to kids of all ages as well as a detailed resources section. Materials also available in Spanish and Chinese.

Cancer in the Family Relief Fund: www.cancerfamilyrelieffund.org
This is a charitable organization that encourages and facilitates grants to children whose parent or guardian is struggling with a diagnosis of cancer. The grants support the children's extracurricular activities while their parent focuses on treatment and recovery. Submit an application online.

Camp Kesem: campkesem.org; (260) 225-3736
Camp Kesem is a free summer camp program for kids whose parents are going through cancer treatment or have passed away from cancer. Run by college students who have gone through specialized training, there are sixty-two chapters in the United States. The camps are one-week "sleep-away" camps for kids age six to sixteen and are held at college campuses.

Kids Konnected: www.kidskonnected.org; (800) 899-2866
Founded by the son of a cancer patient, this nonprofit offers useful tools for parents for talking to kids about cancer, as well as resources for kids and teens. They also hold a free summer camp in California for kids ages seven to thirteen who have had a parent diagnosed with, or lost to, cancer.

Hair and Personal Care
American Cancer Society Wig Bank Line: (877) 227-1596
This program provides free wigs to women in need who have lost their hair due to cancer treatment.

Cancer Be Glammed: www.cancerbeglammed.com
This site is dedicated to non-medical essentials for cancer patients, from bathing suits and pajamas to cancer gift baskets and skin care products. Founded by two women whose lives were directly affected by cancer, their goal is to help patients "recover with dignity, self-esteem, and style."

Chemo Diva Halo Wig: www.chemodiva.com; (813) 451-8401
Chemo Diva is a custom wig maker that uses your own hair. Detailed instructions are on the website; the wig could be covered under your health insurance plan.

DigniCap: www.dignicap.com; (877) 375-8070
This is the only FDA-approved cold cap scalp cooling system. (See Hair: The Bald and the Beautiful in chapter 6 for more on cold caps.) The DigniCap website provides detailed information for both patients and health care providers, including a list of infusion centers that offer the cap.

Look Good Feel Better (LGFB):
www.lookgoodfeelbetter.org, (800) 395-5665
LGFB was founded in 1989 by the Personal Care Products Council Foundation to help cancer patients (women, men, and teenagers) improve their self-confidence while undergoing treatment through group, individual, and self-help sessions for things like skin changes and hair loss. This is a non-branded program affiliated with the American Cancer Society that is staffed by cosmetology professionals who volunteer their time. Go online or call 24 hours a day.

Lymphedivas: www.lymphedivas.com; (866) 411-3482
Started by Rachel Levin Troxell, who passed away from breast cancer, Lymphedivas "provides medically correct fashion for lymphedema" and sell a variety of compression garments for women and men (called Lymphedudes). Rachel's brother, mother, and father (a physician) now run the business in Rachel's memory.

Mondays at Racine: www.mondaysatracine.org; (631) 224-5240
Racine Spa in Islip, New York, provides complimentary salon services to cancer patients every Monday. The cancer care program was created in 2003 by owner Cynthia Sansone and her four sisters, who watched their mom go through cancer treatment. Racine was the inspiration for the Academy Award-nominated short film *Mondays at Racine* (a must-see), which documents cancer patients as they lost their hair during treatment. Racine has inspired many affiliate programs in spas and salons around the United States. Sansone has created a toolkit for other salons to create their own "Mondays," so check with your local beauty salon or spa to see if they offer a similar program or check the Racine website for their "Mondays Salon" listings.

Nearly You: www.nearlyou.com, (866) 722-6168
Nearly You is a source for mastectomy products, including eighty-six types of breast forms, swimsuits, and post-surgical items like camisoles. Their website has detailed measuring guidelines; online and telephone assistance is available.

Pantene Beautiful Lengths: www.pantene.com
Launched in 2006, this program collects real hair to make wigs for female cancer patients. Pantene, a Proctor & Gamble company, partners with the American Cancer Society's Wig Bank Line to distribute the wigs. Go to their website for specifics on how to donate hair or plan your own hair donation event.

Penguin Cold Caps: www.penguincoldcaps.com
A manufacturer of cold caps to help minimize hair loss during treatment (for more information see Hair: The Bald and the Beautiful in chapter 6), Penguin rents caps to patients directly. Telephone customer service is available; see the website for details.

UV Skinz: www.uvskinz.com; (877) UV-SKINZ (887-5469)
This sun protection clothing company was founded by Rhonda Sparks, who lost her young husband to skin cancer. From baby to adult, all of the clothing is SPF50+, the highest level of coverage to protect skin from the sun.

Miscellaneous

CaringBridge: www.caringbridge.org
CaringBridge is a nonprofit that allows people with health issues to create a free website where they can receive donations and well wishes, as well as coordinate assistance with such things as meals. It also includes a journal section for the patient to write a blog. (The sites are ad-free and private.)

Death Over Dinner: www.deathoverdinner.org
This is an organization that helps people have the conversation about how they want to die; in other words, "the most difficult conversation

you will ever avoid." Founded by Michael Hebb, the website gives step-by-step instructions for preparing for a dinner where you do just that, and includes written materials and a video.

Emily McDowell Studio: www.emilymcdowell.com

Artist (and Hodgkin's lymphoma survivor) McDowell founded a stationery and gift company that makes an "empathy card" line of cards you will actually want to send to a cancer patient—and that they will want to receive. Her cards are available through the website and select paper stores.

Lotsa Helping Hands: www.lotsahelpinghands.com

This is an online resource for creating a personal calendar for coordinating meals, household help, and other tasks. Creating a "community" is free, and anyone who joins the community can sign up to help.

MyLifeLine.org

Founded by an ovarian cancer survivor, this nonprofit provides free, private, and personal websites for cancer patients and their caregivers. Patients can set up a page to write updates, create a calendar to schedule help, or set up a donation page to collect funds for treatment.

PillPack: www.Pillpack.com; (855) 745-5725

This is an online, full-service pharmacy based in Manchester, NH, that packages your medications in boxes by time of day, making it easy to organize multiple medications. You pay standard co-pays and shipping is free; they carry most medications as well as over-the-counter products. (Note: they do not fill Schedule II prescriptions.)

Wellist: www.wellist.com; (855) 935-5478

Wellist is a free online resource for cancer patients and their friends and families to get connected to services they need outside of the hospital. They have personalized recommendations for services like meal delivery and home cleaning, as well as supportive services like integrated therapies and support groups. Wellist offers local recommendations in the Greater Boston area and over four hundred different national recommendations. The site also offers a gift registry called a "Wellistry" as a way to let friends and family know how they can support the patient. One hundred percent of all donations go directly to the patients, except for a small processing fee. Wellist also offers live phone and email support.

Fertility Resources
Hope for Two: www.hopefortwo.org; (800) 743-4471
Hope for Two is an international nonprofit dedicated to helping women who are pregnant when they're diagnosed with cancer. The program refers to itself as "The Pregnant with Cancer Network," and provides emotional and educational support.

Inspire: www.inspire.com
Inspire offers online patient communities with support groups for specific cancer patients facing or dealing with infertility.

Livestrong Foundation:
www.livestrong.org/we-can-help/fertility-services
Livestrong offers a variety of fertility services, including lists of fertility centers that provide discounts to cancer patients, donated fertility drugs, and a risk calculator to see how some cancer treatments can affect fertility.

National Comprehensive Cancer Network (NCCN): www.nccn.org
NCCN is a not-for-profit alliance of twenty-six of the top cancer treatment centers dedicated to cancer patient care and research. They offer resources for financial issues, health insurance reimbursement, and treatment education in text and app form, and they created an online "flipbook" that shows fertility preservation options.

Oncofertility Consortium: www.oncofertility.northwestern.edu
This site provides a list of adoption agencies that will work with couples with a cancer history.

Save My Fertility: www.savemyfertility.org
This is a website and iPhone app that has extensive information for men and women facing cancer-related fertility issues as well as parents of children who have been diagnosed with cancer. Established in 1997 by the Endocrine Society.

Crowdfunding Websites

Note: All of the crowdfunding websites listed here allow you to set up pages with no fundraising minimums and no deadlines, so the funding sites stay active as long as you need them. They also offer mobile apps so you can track funding and donate through your cell phone.

CrowdRise: www.crowdrise.com
CrowdRise allows individuals and nonprofits to set up free crowdfunding website pages. They charge a total fee of 3 percent for all donations.

GoFundMe: www.gofundme.com
This is an online fundraising site that takes approximately 8 percent of each donation you receive.

IndieGoGo: www.indiegogo.com
IndieGoGo is an international crowdfunding site, and charges 5 percent of the total funds raised.

YouCaring: www.youcaring.com
As a "compassionate crowdfunding" site, YouCaring doesn't charge a fee for funds raised through a campaign; the only fees are charged by PayPal.

Local Service Organizations

Local service or volunteer organizations such as Catholic Charities USA and Jewish Social Services may offer financial assistance and meal delivery or food pantry assistance. Some of these organizations offer grants to help cover the cost of cancer treatment, and others provide assistance with specific services such as travel or medications.

General assistance programs providing food, housing, and other services may be available from your county or city department of social services. Many cities have emergency funds, either specifically for cancer patients or anyone with a serious illness. Check with your city for more information.

Travel and Temporary Housing Assistance

Air Care Alliance (ACA): www.aircarealliance.org; (888) 260-9707
This organization maintains a list of free transportation services provided by volunteer pilots and charitable aviation groups.

Air Charity Network: www.aircharitynetwork.org; (877) 621-7177
This organization coordinates free air transportation in unpressurized small aircraft for people in need through a network of volunteer pilots in the United States.

Corporate Angel Network:
www.corpangelnetwork.org, (866) 328-1313
This group arranges free air transportation for cancer patients and bone marrow recipients and donors traveling to treatment using empty seats on corporate jets. (A family member can travel with you.) Register online within three weeks of your medical appointment to request flights.

Footprints in the Sky: www.footprintsflights.org; (303) 799-0461
This Denver-based nonprofit, founded by pilot Johnny Langland, provides free transportation to patients and their family members or a caregiver on corporate or private planes. Fill out a flight request form online; there is a $35 application fee.

Healthcare Hospitality Network, Inc. (HHN):
www.hhnetwork.org, (800) 542-9730
HHN is an association of two hundred nonprofit organizations that provide lodging and support services to families and their loved ones who are receiving medical treatment away from home.

Hope Lodge: www.cancer.org/treatment/
supportprogramsservices/hopelodge, (800) 227-2345
Operated by the American Cancer Society, Hope Lodge gives cancer patients and their caregivers a free place to stay while receiving treatment in another city. Currently there are thirty-one Hope Lodge locations throughout the United States.

Joe's House: www.joeshouse.org; (877) 563-7468
Joe's House is a nonprofit that offers a "lodging guide for cancer patients" and includes a list of discounted hotels and motels.

LifeLine Pilots: www.lifelinepilots.org; (800) 822-7972
Through LifeLine Pilots, volunteer pilots donate their time and all flight expenses to people in need of free transportation for ongoing treatment, diagnosis, and follow-up care. Request flights and submit the application on their website.

Mercy Medical Angels (MMA):
mercymedical.org, (888) 675-1805, (757) 318-9174
A "charitable medical tranportation system," MMA coordinates various forms of transportation for patients in need, including flights and ground transportation. They work with, and administer, several patient flight services.

National Patient Travel Center:
www.patienttravel.org, (800) 296-1217
This resource provides information about long-distance travel for cancer patients and their families in need of travel assistance.

Patient AirLift Services (PALS): www.palservices.org; (888) 818-1231
PALS is a nonprofit network, established in 2010, of volunteer pilots who
provide air transportation at no cost to individuals in need of diagnosis,
treatment, or follow-up or other compassionate or humanitarian reasons.
Based in New York, they have provided over ten thousand free flights
since they began.

Research Foundations
Breast Cancer Research Foundation (BCRF):
www.bcrfcure.org, (866) 346-3228
This nonprofit funds breast cancer research—to over 200 researchers—as
well as sponsoring awareness programs. A reliable source for current
breast cancer research.

Cycle for Survival: www.cycleforsurvival.com
This nonprofit raises research money for rare cancers (types of cancer
that affect fewer than 200,000 people in the United States, according
to the NIH). They hold annual spin cycle events in February and March;
all the money raised goes directly to Memorial Sloan Kettering Cancer
Center in New York City for cancer research.

The Jimmy Fund: www.jimmyfund.org
This foundation raises money for Boston's Dana-Farber Cancer Institute
to fund adult and pediatric cancer care and research, including clinical
trials and patient survivorship programs.

The Laura Mercier Ovarian Cancer Fund (LMOCF):
lauramercierovariancancerfund.org
Started in 2012 by co-founder Laura Mercier and president and CEO
Claudia Poccia, this nonprofit fund supports research and education for
ovarian cancer patients and women at risk for the disease. The company
also donates 100 percent of the profits from certain Laura Mercier brand
beauty products to the fund, which also works with nonprofits in the
United Kingdom, Canada, and France.

Ovarian Cancer Research Fund Alliance (OCRFA): www.ocrfa.org, (212) 268-1002

The mission of this nonprofit (a newly formed organization, combining the Ovarian Cancer Research Fund and the Ovarian Cancer National Alliance) is to treat and prevent ovarian cancer as well as fund research. They offer educational materials in both English and Spanish and the website offers a community "wall" of survivor stories and tributes. They also hold fundraising and community events around the United States to fund their research grants.

Breast Cancer Organizations

African American Breast Care Alliance: aabcainc.org; (612) 825-3675

This organization provides social, emotional, and educational support for African American breast cancer patients.

Breast Cancer Action (BCA): www.bcaction.org, (877) 2-STOPBC (877-278-6722) or (415) 243-4301

A nonprofit advocacy group based in San Francisco, BCA focuses on "health justice" and ending the "breast cancer epidemic." They provide a wide range of resources and education for breast cancer patients.

Bright Pink: www.brightpink.org

This nonprofit is dedicated to early prevention of breast and ovarian cancer. They provide mentor "PinkPals," outreach groups, and educational materials to medical schools.

The Carey Foundation: www.careyfoundation.org

Started by cancer patient Linda Carey and her husband Bob, this foundation is devoted to providing female and male breast cancer patients, survivors, and their families with financial assistance. The money raised by the foundation is given through grants to organizations that distribute it directly to those in need to cover costs not covered by health insurance, such as child care and transportation. The Careys also founded The Tutu Project (www.thetutuproject.com), which promotes breast cancer awareness and helps fund the Carey Foundation.

Comadre a Comadre Project: www.comadre.unm.edu; (505) 277-0111
This is a program for Hispanic/Latina breast cancer patients and their
caregivers that is run out of the University of New Mexico in Albuquerque.
They provide educational materials, connect patients with services and
resources, and provide peer and group support. Materials and support
available in English and Spanish.

For3Sisters: www.for3sisters.com
This is an organization that was founded by a firefighter who lost three
sisters to breast cancer. It provides education and programs with direct
resources for female and male breast cancer patients. Apply online.

Living Beyond Breast Cancer (LBBC):
www.lbbc.org, (855) 807-6386
LBBC is a nonprofit that provides support and information for breast cancer patients. They offer a telephone help line, webinars, conferences, and
specialized programs such as the Young Women's Initiative for patients
diagnosed under the age of forty-five.

Sharsheret: www.sharsheret.org; (866) 474-2774
Sharsheret is a nonprofit founded by a breast cancer patient that offers
resources for young Jewish breast cancer and ovarian cancer patients. A
wide variety of resources for patients at every stage, including education,
online live chat support, and support for caregivers and family members.

Tigerlily Foundation: www.tigerlilyfoundation.org; (888) 580-6253
This is a nonprofit based in Virginia and founded by breast cancer survivor Maimah Karmo to assist the young adult breast cancer population
(ages fifteen to forty). Education, advocacy, support, and empowerment
are the goals; more information and resources are on their website.

Triple Negative Breast Cancer (TNBC) Foundation:
www.tnbcfoundation.org, (877) 880-8622
TNBC Foundation is a nonprofit specifically for triple-negative breast
cancer patients with a commitment to research and patient education,
including clinical trial information and caregiver and patient information
for certain at-risk groups.

Young Survival Coalition (YSC): www.youngsurvival.org; (877) 972-1011
YSC is a nonprofit that provides information and support to women under forty who are at risk, have been diagnosed with, or are survivors of breast cancer. YSC offers a wide range of information, programs, and fundraisers around the United States.

Zero Breast Cancer: www.zerobreastcancer.org
This is a community-based nonprofit in Northern California that is dedicated to research and the environmental causes of breast cancer. Educational and research materials are available.

Just for Fun

Hopefully you can insert a little bit of fun in this road trip and find a retreat or adventure to participate in, whether you're in treatment or a thriving survivor. Check out these (mostly) free programs devoted to cancer patients and/or their families. Also ask your medical center or hospital; they sometimes offer their own retreats.

Athletes 4 Cancer: www.athletes4cancer.org; (415) 617-5678
Based in Oregon, this nonprofit offers snow and sea athletic retreats for cancer patients ages eighteen to thirty-nine in Mount Hood, Oregon, and Maui, Hawaii, as well as a survivor retreat in Oregon. Patients must be finished with active treatment at least three months before the start date of the program. The camp is free but travel costs are not covered. Apply online.

Big Sky Yoga Retreats – Cowgirls vs. Cancer:
www.bigskyyogaretreats.com, (406) 219-7685
This program is an annual retreat in Clyde Park, Montana, for breast cancer patients and survivors. The four–day retreat combines horsemanship, yoga, and "holistic healing." Participants are chosen through a nomination process; check the website for details.

Camp Mak-A-Dream: www.campdream.org; (406) 549-5987
Provides a variety of free, year-round camps and programs on a 87 acre ranch in Montana for cancer patients and their siblings. All programs are medically supervised and are offered for kids, teens, young adults, and adults. Travel costs are not included but a limited number of travel scholarships available to qualified applicants. Apply online.

Casting for Recovery: castingforrecovery.org
This group offers free weekend fly-fishing retreats for female breast cancer patients from April through November, with different regions available. Interested patients should apply online, and participants are chosen via a lottery system.

Epic Experience: www.EpicExperience.org; (855) 650-9907
This nonprofit, based in Colorado, provides adult weeklong wilderness adventures for adult cancer patients ages eighteen and over. Apply online.

First Descents: www.firstdescents.org
First Descents's Out Living It Project offers free adventure camps for young cancer patients (ages eighteen to thirty-nine; you must have been at least fifteen years old at time of diagnosis). Locations around the United States; apply online (travel scholarships are also available for qualified applicants). They also offer specialty options like a "40+" program for survivors ages forty through forty-nine.

Little Pink Houses of Hope: www.littlepink.org
This nonprofit provides vacation houses for breast cancer patients and their families (as well as some couples-only options). The houses are located throughout the United States and patients apply a year ahead. It's a free weeklong vacation—it's worth an application! Apply online.

Live by Living: www.livebyliving.org; (303) 808-2339
This group offers all cancer patients, survivors, and their caregivers organized day hikes and walks as well as overnight hiking and camping trips in Colorado. All programs are free; register online.

Pink Lemonade Project: pinklemonadeproject.org
This organization offers retreats for breast cancer survivors and retreats for survivors and their partners. Retreats are staffed by oncology social workers in Washington state and are free of charge, but travel expenses are not covered; apply online.

Reel Recovery: www.reelrecovery.net; (800) 699-4490
This is an organization that provides fly-fishing retreats in various locations to men age twenty-one and over with any form of cancer (patients or those in remission). The twelve-person retreats are staffed by psychosocial professionals and professional fly fishers; apply through their website. (The retreats are free of charge, but participants cover travel costs.)

Smith Center for Healing and the Arts:
www.smithcenter.org, (202) 483-8600
The Smith Center offers three- and seven-day retreats just outside their headquarters in Washington, DC. Workshops and one-day retreats are also offered in their offices. Retreats are staffed by licensed psychotherapists. All cancer patients, including those in remission, are welcome to apply.

Stowe Weekend of Hope: www.stowehope.org
This is an annual event held in Stowe, Vermont, for all cancer patients and survivors. Lectures by oncologists discussing the latest cancer findings, art and wellness workshops, hikes, and yoga are offered. First-time attendees attend for free, including lodging (except for a processing fee). Register online; held annually the first weekend in May.

True North Treks: www.truenorthtreks.org; (773) 972-2367
Based in Illinois, True North is a nonprofit that offers free retreats for young adult cancer survivors. Survivors as well as caregivers/spouses are eligible for mini- and week-long retreats held throughout the United States. Apply online.

ACKNOWLEDGMENTS

The list of people who helped me—and continue to help me—stay alive could fill a book, but I'll try and list them all here. I am profoundly grateful to each and every one of you.

Thanks to:

- First, to my family: my husband Munir and our extraordinary kids, Penelope and Roman; my sister Lesley, my brother-in-law Tim, and my sweet, smart, and caring nieces, Caroline, Kendall, and Colette; my dad, Stephen; my mom, Bernadette; Adam; my aunt Paula, and Joe Coradetti & family;

- To my beloved "aunts": Donna, Ellen L., and Pauline, for too many things to list here;

- To the entire extended Reidy family for their tireless support;

- To Rob and Erin, for making that call;

- To Cathy G., for helping with the kids while I was fighting the fight;

- To the InterWest Partners' team of brilliant minds;

- To Carole, Lee, Brandon, and Amy P., for being there;

- To Sondra, for the incredible food and even more incredible friendship;

- To Nancy, MM, and Todd, for the life-changing phone calls;

- To Claire and Matt, for everything, and more;

- To my "girls": Hannah, Faun, Barbara, Mia, Ellen, Beverley, Veronica, Vicki, Joni, and Maria;

- To my brilliant doctors and surgeons, including Dr. Mark Moasser, Dr. Mihaela Cristea, Dr. Robert Foster, Dr. Cheryl Ewing, and Dr. Lee-may Chen;

- To Dr. Vicente Valero and his team at MD Anderson;

- To Dr. Francine Halberg, for such compassionate and brilliant care, and your amazing team: Jana, Jane, Michael, Joe, Shauntel, James, Aron, and Eileen;

- To Dr. Laura Esserman, for your dedication to fighting breast cancer and for eliminating my pain;

- To Dr. Leah Kelley, Dr. Danielle Walker, and Dr. Kara Reinke for getting me through the first few weeks;

- To the incredible nurses who gave me such caring support, in particular Jana, Mary, and Janet T.;

- To Dr. Alan Ashworth, for your unparalleled contribution to breast cancer research and your kind words;

- To Dr. Julie Wolfson-Hackman, for your smiling face, insight, and companionship during the long days at City of Hope;

- To Dr. Jane Jaroszewksi, for your insights and edits to the manuscript;

- To the staff at Marin General Center for Integrative Health and Wellness for your ongoing care and support;

- To Dr. Laura D., for your listening ear;

- To Blue Shield of California;

- To the "Lotsa" community: Kristin, Kerry, Mary, Katherine, Carrie, Karin, Ally K., Betsy, Laurie, Kimberly, Barbara G., Susan, Gretchen, Laura R., Alison C., Alexandra, and each and every one of you who dropped off meals and diapers and care packages and cards and/ or sent food and made our family able to function in the midst of the road trip;

- To Kate T., for the laughs, insight, and wisdom, and for believing in this book from day one;

- To Donal Brown, for shaping me as a writer;

- To my Lucas Valley community (and the Lucas Valley Literary Ladies) for your support, school pick-ups, friend- ship, and laughter;

- To Cary, for, among other things, your indefatigable spirit, ongoing support, and the introduction to emojis;

- To Cam M., for your healing Reiki hands;

- To Ranwa and Ed, for your compassion;

- To Dan, for the airline miles and your generosity of spirit;

- To Ed and Theresa, for your encouragement, laughter, ping-pong, and champagne;

- To Cyrus and Amy, for the scientific explanations, beach walks, wine, and coffee;

- To photographers Stephanie Mohan, Lisa Leigh, Alex Tehrani, and Christina McPherson for capturing the before, during, and after;

- To my survivor-thrivers: Katie S., Sally J., Julie V., Amy C., Julie S., Rebecca, Kim, Susan, Happy, Hilary H., Pamela, and Kevin as well as the 2014 "To Celebrate Life" models—to life!

- To Debra Campo, for your soulful, kind words and caring spirit;

- To Gretchen and Clark, for your friendship and so much else;

- To Tara and Ken, for the insight, edits, and doughnuts;

- To Joan N., who I still haven't met in person but who never stopped rooting for me;

- To Mary Woodard Lasker, "the fairy godmother of medical research," according to *BusinessWeek* magazine, who spearheaded the effort for funding cancer research in 1943;

- To Elizabeth Ann "Betty" Ford, who went public with the news of her radical mastectomy in 1974 and brought the words "breast cancer" out in the open;

- To my thoughtful, whip-smart, and encouraging editor Stephanie Knapp, and the amazing team at Seal Press: associate publisher Donna Galassi, who saw the potential in this book from the beginning; the fantastic, eagle-eye copyeditor Holly Cooper who makes me look so smart; Erin Seaward-Hiatt for the stunning book cover; to Barrett Briske, proofreader extraordinaire; designer Domini Dragoone; Molly Conway, for making things happen; and Eva Zimmerman for her support and creative publicity ideas;

- To my brilliant agent Danielle Svetcov, for helping this book come to life;

- And finally, to Sisi D. and Elle S., who made that first appointment at UCSF and opened the door to a treatment—and a life—for me.

APPENDIX

Allison, MD, Kimberly. *Red Sunshine: A Story of Strength and Inspiration from a Doctor Who Survived Stage 3 Breast Cancer*. New York: Penguin Random House, 2011.

Bazell, Robert. *Her-2: The Making of Herceptin, a Revolutionary Treatment for Breast Cancer*. New York: Random House, 1998.

Davis, Devra. *The Secret History of the War on Cancer*. New York: Basic Books, 2007.

Davies, Kevin and Michael White. *Breakthrough: The Race to Find the Breast Cancer Gene*. New York: John Wiley & Sons, Inc., 1995.

DeVita, Jr., MD, Vincent T., and Elizabeth DeVita-Raeburn. *The Death of Cancer: After Fifty Years on the Front Lines of Medicine, a Pioneering Oncologist Reveals Why the War on Cancer Is Winnable—and How We Can Get There*. New York: Farrar, Straus, and Giroux, 2015.

Goodman, Barak, and Ken Burns. *Cancer: The Emperor of All Maladies*. PBS, 2015.

Gubar, Susan. *Memoir of a Debulked Woman: Enduring Ovarian Cancer*. New York: W. W. Norton & Company, 2012.

Harpham, MD, Wendy S. *When a Parent Has Cancer: A Guide to Caring For Your Children*. New York: William Morrow, 2004.

Hodge, Alice and Mary Lonergan. *Taking Charge of Your Health: Understanding the System Could Save Your Life*. Oregon: BookPartners, 1999.

Hoffman, Alice. *Survival Lessons*. Chapel Hill, NC: Algonquin Books of Chapel Hill, 2013.

Holland, MD, Jimmie C. and Sheldon Lewis. *The Human Side of Cancer: Living with Hope, Coping with Uncertainty*. New York: HarperCollins Publishers, 2000.

Hunsicker, Jackson, editor. *Turning Heads: Portraits of Grace, Inspiration, and Possibilities*. Sherman Oaks, CA: Press on Regardless, 2006.

Karp, Nina Montée and Joyce Ostin. *Breast Cancer: The Path of Wellness & Healing*. Montée Productions, 2009.

Kübler-Ross, Elisabeth. *On Death and Dying*. New York: Scribner, 1997.

Kübler-Ross, Elisabeth and David Kessler. *On Grief and Grieving: Finding the Meaning of Grief Through the Five Stages of Loss*. New York: Scribner, 1997.

Lang, Susan S. and Richard B. Patt, MD. *You Don't Have to Suffer: A Complete Guide to Relieving Cancer Pain for Patients and Their Families*. Oxford University Press, 1995.

Linden, David J. *Touch: The Science of Hand, Heart, and Mind*. New York: Viking Press, 2015.

Love, MD, MBA, Susan M. *Dr. Susan Love's Breast Book*. New York: Da Capo Press, 2015 (Sixth Edition).

Malmo, Katherine. *Who in This Room: the Realities of Cancer, Fish, and Demolition*. CALYX Books, 2011.

Mukherjee, MD, Siddhartha. *The Emperor of All Maladies: A Biography of Cancer*. New York: Scribner, 2010.

National Breast Cancer Foundation. "Triple Negative Breast Cancer." www.nationalbreastcancer.org/triple-negative-breast cancer.

Patient Resource Network. "Patient Resource Guide to Understanding Clinical Trials, 2nd edition." PRP Patient Resource Publishing, 2015, www.patientresource.com.

Pogrebin, Letty Cottin. *How to Be a Friend to a Friend Who's Sick*. New York: PublicAffairs, 2013.

Port, MD, Elisa. *The New Generation Breast Cancer Book: How to Navigate Your Diagnosis and Treatment Options—and Remain Optimistic—in an Age of Information Overload*. New York: Ballantine Books, 2015.

Rauch, MD, Paula K. and Anna C. Muriel, MD. *Raising an Emotionally Healthy Child When a Parent is Sick*. McGraw-Hill Education, 2006.

Schreiber-Servan, MD, David. *Anticancer: A New Way of Life*. New York: Viking, 2009.

Skloot, Rebecca. *The Immortal Life of Henrietta Lacks*. New York: Broadway Books, 2010.

Sontag, Susan. *Illness as Metaphor*. New York: Farrar, Straus, and Giroux, 1978.

Trillin, Calvin. *About Alice*. New York: Random House, 2006.

"Understanding Inflammatory Breast Cancer." Houston: The University of Texas MD Anderson Cancer Center; Phyllis Pittman Communications, LTD., 2010.

Wade, Cynthia. *Mondays at Racine*. Cynthia Wade Productions and HBO Documentary, 2012.

Williams, Florence. *Breasts: A Natural and Unnatural History*. New York: W.W. Norton & Company, Inc., 2012.

Van Deernoot, Peter. *Helping Your Children Cope with Your Cancer: A Guide for Parents and Families (Revised Edition)*. New York: Hatherleigh Press, 2005.

INDEX

ABOUT
THE AUTHOR

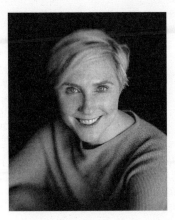

Laura Holmes Haddad is a writer from the San Francisco Bay Area. She received her BA from Smith College and then completed the chef's program at the California Culinary Academy to pursue a career in wine and food writing. Laura spent four years as an assistant cookbook editor at Simon & Schuster before becoming a freelance writer, writing for various websites and magazines and co-authoring and editing cookbooks and lifestyle titles.

In 2012 Laura was diagnosed with Stage IV inflammatory breast cancer at the age of thirty-seven. She is currently in remission. When she's not paddle boarding or swinging on a rope swing with her kids, Laura spends her time writing, blogging, reading, and advocating for young adult cancer patients.

She lives in Northern California with her husband, daughter, son, and a Dalmatian. For more information, visit her website: www.lauraholmeshaddad.com.

Selected Titles from Seal Press

Yogalosophy for Inner Strength: 12 Weeks to Heal Your Heart and Embrace Joy, by Mandy Ingber, $24, 978-1-58005-593-2. Building on the concepts in her New York Times best-selling book Yogalosophy, Mandy Ingber, fitness and wellness instructor to the stars, now gives us a revolutionary and inspiring self-care program to uplift and strengthen the alignment of mind, body, heart, and spirit during times of adversity like loss, transition, grief, or heartbreak.

Mary Jane: The Complete Marijuana Handbook for Women, by Cheri Sicard. $18.00, 978-1-58005-551-2. Mary Jane is a comprehensive guide for women through the wonderful world of weed, dispelling myths and misinformation in a fun, friendly, and frank way.

What You Can When You Can: Healthy Living on Your Terms, by Roni Noone and Carla Birnberg. $14.00, 978-1-58005-573-4. This companion book to the #wycwyc movement teaches you how to harness the power of small steps to achieve your goals for healthier living.

Rocking the Pink: Finding Myself on the Other Side of Cancer, by Laura Roppé. $17.00, 978-1-58005-417-1. The funny, poignant, and inspirational memoir of a woman who took on breast cancer by channeling her inner rock star.

Pale Girl Speaks: A Year Uncovered, by Hillary Fogelson. $16.00, 978-1-58005-444-7. An edgy, funny memoir about a woman who became angry and self-absorbed when she was diagnosed with melanoma—until her father was diagnosed with the same skin cancer, and she had to learn to lead by example and let go of her fear.

Super You: Release Your Inner Superhero, by Emily V. Gordon. $16.00, 978-1-58005-575-8. Super You explores comic book tropes that readers can apply to their own lives to overcome adversity and transform into the best version of themselves.

Find Seal Press Online
sealpress.com
@sealpress
Facebook | Twitter | Instagram | Tumblr | Pinterest